Gastrointestinal Stromal Tumor

Yukinori Kurokawa • Yoshito Komatsu
Editors

Gastrointestinal Stromal Tumor

Research and Practice

Springer

Editors
Yukinori Kurokawa
Department of Gastroenterological Surgery
Osaka University Graduate School
of Medicine
Osaka
Japan

Yoshito Komatsu
Department of Cancer Chemotherapy
Hokkaido University Hospital
Cancer Center
Sapporo
Hokkaido
Japan

ISBN 978-981-13-3205-0 ISBN 978-981-13-3206-7 (eBook)
https://doi.org/10.1007/978-981-13-3206-7

Library of Congress Control Number: 2018968535

This Springer imprint is published by the registered company Springer Nature Singapore Pte Ltd.
The registered company address is: 152 Beach Road, #21-01/04 Gateway East, Singapore 189721, Singapore

Foreword

It is my great pleasure and honor to write a foreword for *Gastrointestinal Stromal Tumor: Research and Practice*. The book systematically covers a broad spectrum from basic knowledge of Gastrointestinal Stromal Tumor (GIST) including epidemiology and clinical guidelines to the latest subjects of molecular diagnosis and treatment by minimal invasive surgery or new agents. It is important that the book has been planned and written in English by leading emerging Japanese specialists in GIST of the next generation based on their scientific knowledge and clinical experience, and now, finally, it is being published.

GIST is a rare cancer that has several challenges compared with more common cancers. Generally, physicians may have little experience and knowledge about it because of its rarity. Such rare cancer is known to frequently lack diagnostic criteria and guidelines for standard treatment. Patients with a rare cancer also lack disease information and referral centers as well as medical specialists. Consequently, such patients show poorer prognosis than those with more common cancer [1]. Rare cancer really needs a good book that is built upon the latest information on diagnosis and treatment. GIST is a model of medical development in rare cancers in that it has diagnostic criteria, a standard treatment, and established guidelines. Diagnostic criteria and guidelines have been established through medical development of molecularly targeted agents based on elucidation of the molecular mechanisms of GIST. As medical development in this area is advancing daily, diagnosis and treatment may change over time, and we should be keenly sensitive to the latest information. GIST is one such area.

Dr. William Osler once said that the practice of medicine is an art, based on science, and also said that it is easier to buy books than to read them and easier to read them than to absorb them [2]. This book is simple and easy to read, and furthermore, it is well organized. It collects new information on standard therapy and the latest topics of emerging therapy required for clinical practice and scientific research. I am confident that this book will be of great help for young physicians and surgeons who treat GIST patients, to increase their clinical competence and scientific knowledge if they absorb its content thoroughly. It has been said, "To study the phenomena of disease without books is to sail an uncharted sea, while to study books without patients is not to go to sea at all." It is my expectation that the book will provide effective learning for medical professionals through their daily practice, which may result in improvement of GIST patients' outcomes.

Toshirou Nishida
National Cancer Center Hospital
Tokyo, Japan

References

1. Gatta G, Capocaccia R, Botta L, et al. Burden and centralised treatment in Europe of rare tumours: results of RARECAREnet—a population-based study. Lancet Oncol. 2017;18(8):1022–39.
2. Stone MJ. The wisdom of Sir William Osler. Am J Cardiol. 1995;75(4):269–76.

Preface

Gastrointestinal Stromal Tumor (GIST) is the most common mesenchymal neoplasm arising in the gastrointestinal tract. Tyrosine kinase inhibitors such as imatinib are highly effective against GIST, because GIST usually has activating mutations in c-*kit*. This causative gene was originally discovered in 1998 by Seiichi Hirota, a Japanese professor, and since then great advances in diagnosis and treatment have been reported by Japanese investigators.

Fortunately, I have recently had an opportunity as a principal investigator to conduct clinical trials for the treatment of GIST. Through the clinical trials, I noticed that there were many things that even the physicians treating this disease were not aware of. However, there were few textbooks that covered the entire field of GIST from basic to clinical aspects. For that major reason, co-editor Prof. Yoshito Komatsu and I planned to publish this book.

All of the expert authors elucidate cutting-edge knowledge in their fields, focusing particularly on data from Japan. This comprehensive and up-to-date collection provides many benefits not only to the physicians but to the basic researchers and co-medical staff dealing with the treatment of GIST.

I thank Mr. Vinoth Kuppan and Ms. Makie Kambara for their kind help in editing this work. In addition, I am deeply grateful to Ms. Yoko Arai for giving me the invaluable opportunity to publish this important book.

Osaka, Japan Yukinori Kurokawa

Contents

Epidemiology

1

Takahiro Higashi

Abstract

GIST is a rare tumor, but determining its incidence is a challenge. Incidence from prior reports ranges from 0.43 to 2.2 per 100,000, but the reports that examined stomach specimen from autopsy or surgery of other diseases suggest that there may be occult GISTs. The distinction between benign and malignant cases is also ambiguous. Cancer registries may not be a reliable source because many limit the reportability of the tumor into only malignant cases. An analysis using hospital-based cancer registries in Japan suggests that overtly malignant cases are about one third of cases that are considered as at least some malignancy (labeled as /1 or /3 in the behavior code of ICD-O-3). We do not know how many cases are there that are considered as benign. Some summaries of the current status of GIST treatment are provided using the same dataset.

Keywords

Incidence · Cancer registry · Reportability

1.1 Reported Incidence of GIST and Challenge in Its Ascertainment

GIST is known as a rare tumor, but is the most common mesenchymal tumor in the gastrointestinal tract. It is believed that the number of annual incidents is approximately 1–2 per 100,000 [1], but studies report a wide variety of incidents depending on regions and period as in a systematic review by Soreide et al. [2] that showed

T. Higashi (✉)
Center for Cancer Registries, National Cancer Center, Tokyo, Japan
e-mail: thigashi@ncc.go.jp

Y. Kurokawa, Y. Komatsu (eds.), *Gastrointestinal Stromal Tumor*,
https://doi.org/10.1007/978-981-13-3206-7_1

variation from the lowest of 0.43 per 100,000 in Shanxi province in China to the high of 1.9–2.2 per year in Hong Kong and Shanghai areas in China, Taiwan, and Northern Norway. This chapter discusses the epidemiology of GIST having in mind the several factors that can influence the results of the studies.

1.1.1 Challenges in Determining the Incidence

The incidence of GIST is influenced by many factors. First, the disease entity of GIST is relatively new based on the immunohistochemical characterization with receptor tyrosine kinase (KIT) expression reported in 1998 [3]. In an attempt to determine the GIST incidence, many epidemiological studies had to reclassify tumors formerly diagnosed as leiomyomas, leiomyosarcomas, schwannomas, and rhabdomyosarcomas into GIST by re-evaluating the pathological specimens. Availability of past specimen and the immunohistochemical technique to researchers naturally affect the case finding and ascertainment of GIST, and thus the reported incidence rate.

Second, GISTs are often found incidentally during thorough pathological examination of the gastrointestinal tracts removed for other cancers. One study revealed that as high as 35 of 100 patients with gastric cancer who had their whole stomach resected were found with microscopic GISTs [4]. Another study that examined consecutive autopsy cases older than 50 years of age with or without cancer showed 22.5% of the cases had GISTs [5]. Most studies of cancer registries do not report how these GISTs are detected. In Asia, where gastric cancer is frequent [6], GISTs may be more likely to be found incidentally during the examination of surgical specimen than the areas where gastric cancer is less common. Furthermore, recently gained popularity of bariatric surgery to treat obesity using sleeve gastrectomy may increase the chance of incidental detection of asymptomatic GISTs, too [7]. The incidence may also be affected by how thorough surgical specimens are usually examined in a routine practice.

Third, prior reports of incidence are difficult to interpret because most cancer registries only include "malignant" cases. For example, the Surveillance, Epidemiology and End-Result (SEER) registry in the USA includes only cases as defined by the behavioral codes of "/2" or "/3" of the International Classification of Diseases Oncology 3rd edition (ICD-O-3) [8]. However, the distinction between malignant and benign cases is ambiguous for several tumors including GISTs. Many prognostic factors for GISTs helped to identify relatively low-risk and high-risk cases, but it had been well known that even low-risk GISTs have the potential of malignant behavior such as recurrence or metastasis, so we cannot appropriately label any GIST as benign [9, 10]. On the other hand, the World Health Organization (WHO) classification of tumors of the digestive systems (known as the WHO blue book) published in 2010 [11] directs that the behavioral code of the ICD-O should be coded based on the prognostic group based on size of tumor and mitotic counts as reported by Miettinen and Lasota [12]. According to the criteria, good prognostic groups (i.e., prognostic groups 1, 2, 3a) are coded as "/0" (benign), poor prognostic groups (i.e., 3b, 5, 6a, 6b) are coded as "/3" (malignant), and cases that do not fall into either groups (i.e., 4) are coded as "/1" (borderline or uncertain malignant potential). However, as described later in this chapter, these WHO criteria have not yet appeared to be adopted widely.

In summary, the level of malignancy at which the epidemiological studies aimed and level of thoroughness of pathological examination can affect the reported incidence rates. The variation found in a recent systematic review of population-based cohorts and registries may be attributable to either the geographical or ethnic variation of the true disease occurrence, or to the variation in reporting or diagnostic practice across setting or countries.

1.1.2 Dataset Used in This Chapter

Having these limitations in mind, we analyzed the data of GIST cases obtained from the national database of hospital-based cancer registries in Japan. The overview of hospital-based cancer registry is described elsewhere [13]. Briefly, the database compiles cancer registries operated by cancer care hospitals designated by the Ministry of Health, Labor and Welfare, Japan, and also receives data from voluntarily participating hospitals. Like the National Cancer Database compiled by Commission on Cancer of the American College of Surgeons, the national database is, by design, hospital-based, not population-based registry database, but the coverage is from 67% (only designated hospitals) to 75% (including voluntarily participating hospitals) of whole cancer cases in Japan, permitting the description of nationwide picture of the practice. The hospital-based cancer registries follow the national standard data format and registry rules starting in 2007, and collect basic information of all cancer cases provided care at the participating hospitals. For GIST, only overtly "malignant" cases (with the behavioral code of "/3" in ICD-O-3) were registered originally up until 2011, when rule was revised so that cases of borderline malignancy ("/1" in ICD-O-3) were also registered. Therefore, we analyzed 3 year cases 2012–2014 that were started with a treatment at the registering hospitals, including both "borderline" and "malignant" cases. The designation is based on the pathologists' opinion at the registering hospital, and not necessarily concordant to the WHO classifications. Because Japanese population-based cancer registries have been underdeveloped with no mandatory reporting until 2016 cases resulting in suboptimal case coverage. As of 2018, the 2016 data from the population registry is not ready for analysis, so the hospital-based cancer registries were the most comprehensive database available for the nationwide analyses.

In the database, a total of 8972 GIST cases were registered for the 3 years. Among all the GIST cases, 2867 (32% of the whole GIST) were cases with the behavioral code of "/3," labeled as overtly "malignant." Although the distinction between "/1" and "/3" is rather opinion-based with no strict definition, we report these numbers because it may be helpful to provide the readers with the ground to be cautious in interpreting the incidence data from various reports.

If we assume that the case coverage is 75%, the incidence rate of the "malignant" cases is 1.1 per 100,000 in Japan, which stays in the range of the global report [2]. If we include all GIST cases, the incidence is 3.3 per 100,000. "Malignant" GIST consists of 0.73% and 7.9% of all cancer cases in the stomach and small intestine, and 0.49% of all malignancies in gastrointestinal tract. The low proportion in the gastric malignancy may be attributable to the high incidence of gastric cancer in Japan, providing pathologists with a larger number of stomach specimen, which, in turn, leads to larger chance of detecting incidental GISTs.

1.1.3 Age and Sex of Patients

The distribution of age of GIST cases in the hospital-based cancer registry is presented in Table 1.1. The distributions of age groups were not different between the borderline or malignant groups. The majority of the cases occurred in 60 and 70 years of age in both malignant and borderline cases. Some cases are found in children. Although the comorbidity is unknown from the registries, the literature reports that they tend to be part of defined syndromes, such as Carney–Stratakis syndrome [14]. It is also reported that the 85% of the pediatric GISTs lack in KIT and PDGFRA mutation, and most are succinate dehydrogenase (SDH) deficient [15].

Although literature reports no particular sex differences in adult cases, the patients in the Japanese hospital-based registry were 55% male and 45% female. This male preponderance may be because of a detection bias due to the

Table 1.1 Age distribution

	Borderline (/1)		Malignant (/3)	
Age groups	*N*	%	*N*	%
0–29	21	0.4	14	0.5
30–39	136	2.2	74	2.6
40–49	358	5.9	175	6.1
50–59	752	12.3	395	13.8
60–69	1,887	30.9	846	29.5
70–79	2093	34.3	931	32.5
80–89	810	13.3	412	14.4
90–	48	0.8	20	0.7
Total	6105	100.0	2867	100.0

fact that gastric cancer is more common in males than females, and some of the GIST cases are found incidentally and registered based on the borderline histology on a pathological examination of the stomach resected for gastric carcinoma.

1.2 Site of Tumor and Stage Distribution

From now on, we focus on the cases with "/3" behavioral codes. Previous reports state that the most common location of the tumor is stomach (55–60%), followed by small intestine (32–35%). The trend was also found in the Japanese hospital-based registry as shown in Table 1.2. The greater proportion of stomach (66% and 75% in malignancy and borderline cases) may be because of the larger chance of detection of stomach due to the screening programs of gastric cancer through endoscopy and upper gastrointestinal contrast X-ray implemented as publicly funded screening program in Japan.

Few prior studies describe the stage distribution from cancer registries. Although the finding may not be generalizable to other countries or settings, Table 1.3 shows the distribution of stages among cases registered in the Japanese hospital-based registries

Table 1.2 Site distribution

	Borderline (/1)		Malignant (/3)	
Site	*N*	%	*N*	%
Esophagus	84	1.4	33	1.2
Stomach	4582	75.1	1903	66.4
Small intestine	1124	18.4	687	24.0
Colon	49	0.8	27	0.9
Rectum	192	3.1	122	4.3
Other/Unknown	74	1.2	95	3.3
Total	6105	100.0	2867	100.0

Table 1.3 UICC stages ("/3" cases)

	Stomach		Small intestine	
Stage	*N*	%	*N*	%
I	1091	57.3	240	34.9
II	259	13.6	95	13.8
III	268	14.1	195	28.4
IV	162	8.5	118	17.2
Unknown	123	6.5	39	5.7
Total	1903	100.0	687	100.0

according to Union for International Cancer Control (UICC) 7th edition. The stages were based on pathological stages supplemented by clinical stages when pathological stages were not available. More than half of the gastric GIST were Stage I and the majority of the cases in small intestine were Stage I or II. However, substantial proportion (17.2%) of cases in small intestine has either nodal or distant metastasis (Stage IV).

1.3 Treatment Modalities

To date, no study has described the practice patterns, but the national database of hospital-based registries allows us to look at a rough practice patterns, though it captures only treatment provided in the registering facilities. Table 1.4 presents the treatment choice for malignant cases of the stomach and small intestine. The majority (72% of the stomach and 60% of the small intestine) of the patients were treated with surgery only, and 19.5% and 31.3% received surgery and chemotherapy as the first-line therapy. (The timing of chemotherapy (e.g., before or after surgery) is not recorded in the registry.) One fourth of the gastric GIST were treated by chemotherapy with or without surgery.

1.4 Molecular/Genomic Frequencies

Molecular/genomic information were not available in the hospital-based cancer registries, so we must rely on the prior literature for the distribution of molecular markers. Literature shows that most GISTs are immunoreactive for KIT (a receptor tyrosine kinase), but about 5% of the gastric GISTs lacked KIT positivity [16]. Discovered on GIST (DOG1) is another marker that is sensitive and specific to GIST irrespective of KIT status [17–19]. Therefore, this marker can be used to diagnose the GIST that is KIT negative. Given the cost of testing, reports on molecular frequency are usually not population-based, the accurate prevalence of genetic markers remains unknown, making the value of discussion of their epidemiology uncertain. Molecular profiles of GISTs and their characteristics will be discussed in other chapters.

Table 1.4 Therapeutic modalities ("/3" cases)

	Stomach		Small intestine	
Therapy[a]	*N*	%	*N*	%
Surgery only	1364	71.7	411	59.8
Surgery + chemotherapy	371	19.5	215	31.3
Chemotherapy only	94	4.9	44	6.4
Endoscopy	24	1.3	17[b]	2.5[b]
Others	50	2.6		
Total	1903	100.0	687	100.0

[a]Therapy provided in the registering facility as a first-line course
[b]Grouped with "others" because only few cases were treated with endoscopy

1.5 Survival and Predictors of Recurrence

Since the introduction of imatinib dramatically improved the survival of GIST patients [20, 21], the data of natural history of survival based on old data may not be relevant any more. The popular prognosis groupings based on tumor size and mitotic counts are originally derived from pre-imatinib era, but re-evaluated in predicting recurrence probability after surgical removal.

Two most popular grouping are one created by the NIH risk categories created in the consensus report and one using Air Forces Institute of Pathology (AFIP) by Miettinen and colleagues. Both generally say that tumors of ≤2 cm in size or ≤5/50 HPF in mitotic counts have very low risk (or even no risk by AFIP criteria). Table 1.5 portraits the difference in risk categorizations between conventional NIH risk categories, AFIP prognostic groups, the WHO classification of the level of malignancy, and UICC tumor classifications and stages based on the 8th edition. Tumor of 2–5 cm size and mitotic count of 6–10/50 HPF are a major discrepancy of the categorization between NIH risk categories and the newer classifications.

As the imatinib treatment spreads and the adjuvant therapy with imatinib after surgical resection has been shown to reduce the recurrence [22, 23], the risk groups have been applied to identify candidates for adjuvant therapy. Compiling 10 series of population-based studies of operable GIST patients, Joensuu et al. [24] tested the NIH categories, AFIP prognostic groups, and the modifications of NIH categories. A modified NIH classification regrouped cases with tumor ruptures during surgery, the 2–5 cm tumor with 6–10 mitotic count of stomach GIST, and 5–10 cm tumors with <5 mitotic counts of non-gastric GIST into the high-risk group. Overall, the 10- and 20-year recurrence-free survival were 62.9% and 57.3% (taking death without recurrence as censoring) and overall survival were 56.4% and 36.8%. The area under curve statistics to predict 10-year recurrence based on the high-risk

Table 1.5 Different risk grouping based on tumor size and mitotic count

			AFIP				UICC 8th edition classification/stage[a]			
Tumor size	Mitotic count	NIH risk group	Group	Stomach	Small intestine	WHO	T class	G class	Stomach	Small intestine
≤2[b]	≤5	Very low	1	None	None	/0	T1	Low	IA	I
2–5[c]	≤5	Low	2	Very low	Low		T2	Low	IA	I
5–10[c]	≤5	Intermediate	3a	Low	Moderate		T3	Low	IB	II
≤2[b]	6–10		4	[d]	[d]	/1	T1	High	II	IIIA
2–5[c]	6–10		5	Moderate	High	/3	T2	High	II	IIIB
>10	≤5	High	3b	Moderate	High		T4	Low	II	IIIA
2–5[c]	>10		5	Moderate	High		T2	High	II	IIIB
5–10[c]	>5		6a	High	High		T3	High	IIIA	IIIB
>10	>5		6b	High	High		T4	High	IIIB	IIIB

[a]Assuming N0M0
[b]Equal sign does not apply in NIH grouping
[c]Lower boundary is not included in grouping other than NIH
[d]The cell had too few cases to calculate the risk

group was similar among three risk classifications (AUC 0.78–0.82), but the newly created non-linear model, which is expressed in a contour map, had substantially higher AUC (0.87–0.88). Another study conducted in Japan revealed that among the three risk classifications and the American Joint Committee on Cancer (AJCC) stages 7th edition, which is equivalent to UICC stages 7th edition, the high-risk group of modified NIH classification had the greatest sensitivity for recurrence, and the AJCC stages were the highest accuracy [25].

1.6 Summary

Describing the epidemiology of GIST has unique challenge. It is relatively new entity defined by not only microscopic morphology but also molecular/genetic characterization. Incidental discovery in autopsy or surgical specimen was obtained because other diseases are not uncommon. The rigor of pathological examination and availability of molecular/genetic test affect the reported incidence of GISTs. Furthermore, the level of malignancy, which affects the reportability to conventional cancer registries, is described in the WHO classification by prognostic estimation, not solely on pathological findings.

These challenges may be a herald of new era with inevitable transformation of cancer surveillance and epidemiology. For more than a hundred years, cancers were diagnosed based on its microscopic shape. Now "more micro," molecular, characteristics create the disease entity and predict the prognosis. Epidemiology of GIST is a leading case that clearly indicates the need of new perspectives.

References

1. DeMatteo RP, Maki R, Agulnik M, et al. Gastrointestinal stromal tumor. In: AJCC cancer staging manual. Chicago: Springer; 2017.
2. Soreide K, Sandvik OM, Soreide JA, Giljaca V, Jureckova A, Bulusu VR. Global epidemiology of gastrointestinal stromal tumours (GIST): a systematic review of population-based cohort studies. Cancer Epidemiol. 2016;40:39–46.
3. Hirota S, Isozaki K, Moriyama Y, et al. Gain-of-function mutations of c-kit in human gastrointestinal stromal tumors. Science. 1998;279:577–80.
4. Kawanowa K, Sakuma Y, Sakurai S, et al. High incidence of microscopic gastrointestinal stromal tumors in the stomach. Hum Pathol. 2006;37:1527–35.
5. Agaimy A, Wunsch PH, Hofstaedter F, et al. Minute gastric sclerosing stromal tumors (GIST tumorlets) are common in adults and frequently show c-KIT mutations. Am J Surg Pathol. 2007;31:113–20.
6. Global Cancer Observatory. 2012. https://gco.iarc.fr/. Accessed 1 May 2018.
7. Estimate of Bariatric Surgery Numbers, 2011-2016. 2018. https://asmbs.org/resources/estimate-of-bariatric-surgery-numbers. Accessed 1 May 2018.
8. SEER. Program coding and staging manual 2016. 2016. https://seer.cancer.gov/manuals/2016/SPCSM_2016_maindoc.pdf. Accessed 1 May 2018.
9. Rubin BP, Fletcher JA, Fletcher CD. Molecular insights into the histogenesis and pathogenesis of gastrointestinal stromal tumors. Int J Surg Pathol. 2000;8:5–10.

10. Fletcher CD, Berman JJ, Corless C, et al. Diagnosis of gastrointestinal stromal tumors: a consensus approach. Hum Pathol. 2002;33:459–65.
11. Miettinen MM, Lasota J, Coless CL, et al. Gastrointestinal stromal tumours. In: WHO classification of tumours of the digestive system. 4th ed. Geneva: World Health Organization; 2010.
12. Miettinen M, Lasota J. Gastrointestinal stromal tumors: pathology and prognosis at different sites. Semin Diagn Pathol. 2006;23:70–83.
13. Higashi T, Nakamura F, Shibata A, Emori Y, Nishimoto H. The national database of hospital-based cancer registries: a nationwide infrastructure to support evidence-based cancer care and cancer control policy in Japan. Jpn J Clin Oncol. 2014;44:2–8.
14. Pappo AS, Janeway KA. Pediatric gastrointestinal stromal tumors. Hematol Oncol Clin North Am. 2009;23:15–34, vii.
15. Janeway KA, Kim SY, Lodish M, et al. Defects in succinate dehydrogenase in gastrointestinal stromal tumors lacking KIT and PDGFRA mutations. Proc Natl Acad Sci U S A. 2011;108:314–8.
16. Medeiros F, Corless CL, Duensing A, et al. KIT-negative gastrointestinal stromal tumors: proof of concept and therapeutic implications. Am J Surg Pathol. 2004;28:889–94.
17. Espinosa I, Lee CH, Kim MK, et al. A novel monoclonal antibody against DOG1 is a sensitive and specific marker for gastrointestinal stromal tumors. Am J Surg Pathol. 2008;32:210–8.
18. Lopes LF, West RB, Bacchi LM, van de Rijn M, Bacchi CE. DOG1 for the diagnosis of gastrointestinal stromal tumor (GIST): Comparison between 2 different antibodies. Appl Immunohistochem Mol Morphol. 2010;18:333–7.
19. West RB, Corless CL, Chen X, et al. The novel marker, DOG1, is expressed ubiquitously in gastrointestinal stromal tumors irrespective of KIT or PDGFRA mutation status. Am J Pathol. 2004;165:107–13.
20. Perez EA, Livingstone AS, Franceschi D, et al. Current incidence and outcomes of gastrointestinal mesenchymal tumors including gastrointestinal stromal tumors. J Am Coll Surg. 2006;202:623–9.
21. Chiang NJ, Chen LT, Tsai CR, Chang JS. The epidemiology of gastrointestinal stromal tumors in Taiwan, 1998-2008: a nation-wide cancer registry-based study. BMC Cancer. 2014;14:102.
22. Dematteo RP, Ballman KV, Antonescu CR, et al. Adjuvant imatinib mesylate after resection of localised, primary gastrointestinal stromal tumour: a randomised, double-blind, placebo-controlled trial. Lancet. 2009;373:1097–104.
23. Joensuu H, Eriksson M, Sundby Hall K, et al. One vs three years of adjuvant imatinib for operable gastrointestinal stromal tumor: a randomized trial. JAMA. 2012;307:1265–72.
24. Joensuu H, Vehtari A, Riihimaki J, et al. Risk of recurrence of gastrointestinal stromal tumour after surgery: an analysis of pooled population-based cohorts. Lancet Oncol. 2012;13:265–74.
25. Yanagimoto Y, Takahashi T, Muguruma K, et al. Re-appraisal of risk classifications for primary gastrointestinal stromal tumors (GISTs) after complete resection: indications for adjuvant therapy. Gastric Cancer. 2015;18:426–33.

Histology

2

Hidetaka Yamamoto

Abstract

The discovery of *KIT* gene mutation in gastrointestinal stromal tumor (GIST) has provided a paradigm shift in the classification, diagnosis, and molecular-targeted therapy of gastrointestinal mesenchymal tumors. According to a recent concept, GIST is considered a spindle or epithelioid cell neoplasm which basically expresses KIT protein and has *KIT* or *platelet-derived growth factor receptor-alpha (PDGFRA)* gene mutation. Exceptional cases are immunohistochemically negative or weakly positive for KIT (often with *PDGFRA* mutation), and minor subset has another gene alteration such as *succinate dehydrogenase (SDH), RAS, NF1,* or *BRAF*. There are growing evidences of phenotype–genotype correlations in GIST. Risk stratification based on mitotic counts, tumor size, and rupture is useful for the prognostication and management of patients with GIST. GISTs should be distinguished from various types of neoplasms such as leiomyoma, schwannoma, and inflammatory myofibroblastic tumor, although leiomyosarcoma of the gastrointestinal tract has become a very rare entity in the "KIT" era. Both histopathological procedures and molecular investigations are important for the evolution of diagnosis and treatment of GIST and mimics.

Keywords

Gastrointestinal stromal tumor · Histology · Genotype · Immunohistochemistry · Succinate dehydrogenase

H. Yamamoto (✉)
Department of Pathology, Kyushu University Hospital, Fukuoka, Japan

Department of Anatomic Pathology, Kyushu University Graduate School of Medicine, Fukuoka, Japan
e-mail: hidetaka@surgpath.med.kyushu-u.ac.jp

Y. Kurokawa, Y. Komatsu (eds.), *Gastrointestinal Stromal Tumor*,
https://doi.org/10.1007/978-981-13-3206-7_2

2.1 The Definition of GIST

Before the discovery of the oncogenic role of *KIT* gene mutation in GISTs by Hirota et al. in 1998 [1], most GISTs were lumped into the category of smooth muscle tumors or neurogenic tumors. For example, most high-grade GISTs were diagnosed as "leiomyosarcoma" and low-grade GISTs were included in "leiomyoma." Epithelioid GISTs were diagnosed as "epithelioid leiomyosarcoma," "malignant leiomyoblastoma," or "leiomyoblastoma" based on cellular atypia and mitotic activity; however, the pathological diagnoses were often arbitrary. In the "KIT" era, GIST has become the most common mesenchymal tumor of the gastrointestinal (GI) tract [2, 3]. According to a recent concept, GIST is considered a spindle or epithelioid cell neoplasm which typically expresses KIT protein and has *KIT* or *platelet-derived growth factor receptor-alpha (PDGFRA)* gene mutation [2–4]. Exceptional cases are immunohistochemically negative or weakly positive for KIT (often with *PDGFRA* mutation), and minor subset has another gene alteration such as *succinate dehydrogenase (SDH), RAS, NF1,* or *BRAF* [4, 5].

Since therapeutic effect of tyrosine kinase inhibitor for clinically malignant and high-risk GISTs was confirmed by several clinical studies, GISTs have served as an excellent model for the molecular-based classification, diagnosis, and therapy of malignant tumors, because KIT is not only a diagnostic marker but also an oncogenic driver and therapeutic target.

2.2 Histopathological Features of GIST

Clinicopathological and genetic features of GISTs are summarized in Table 2.1. Most patients with GISTs are middle-aged to elderly adults, and pediatric cases are very rare. The stomach is the most common site of GISTs, followed by the small intestine. Colorectal and esophageal primary tumors are rare.

Macroscopically, most GISTs present as submucosal tumor, varying from minimal mural nodule to large mass, occasionally accompanied by mucosal ulcer and tumor rupture. On the cut-surface, GISTs vary in color from pale to pink tan, accompanied by various degrees of hemorrhage, necrosis, and cystic change [4]. Myxoid change is often seen in gastric GIST with *PDGFRA* mutation.

The normal counterpart of GIST is believed to be the interstitial cell of Cajal (ICC), which is the KIT/CD34-positive pacemaker cell located at the Auerbach's plexus in the muscularis propria of GI tract wall. This idea is supported by the fact that most small GISTs have connection with muscularis propria of GI tract wall.

Histologically, GIST is roughly classified as spindle cell type, epithelioid cell type, or mixed spindle/epithelioid cell type (Fig. 2.1). Miettinen and Lasota have described the further cytological subtypes of gastric GIST as follows: sclerosing spindle cell, palisading-vacuolated spindle cell, hypercellular spindle cell, sarcomatous spindle cell, sclerosing epithelioid cell, dyscohesive epithelioid cell, hypercellular epithelioid cell, and sarcomatous epithelioid cell [2]. Among these subtypes, the sarcomatous spindle cell and sarcomatous epithelioid cell subtypes are characterized by plump and hyperchromatic nuclei, and are usually mitotically active with aggressive behavior. In contrast, sclerosing spindle cell subtype usually shows low

Table 2.1 Summary of GIST variants and clinicopathological and genetic features

GIST subtype	Age (year)	Sex	Site	Multiplicity	Cell type	Genotype
Sporadic, conventional	>40	M, F	Stomach, small intestine	No	Spi, Epi, Mix	KIT, PDGFRA
			>Esophagus, colorectum, omentum, mesentery			Rare; BRAF, RAS, PIK3CA
KIT-negative	>40	M, F	Stomach, omentum	No	Epi, Mix	PDGFRA
Pediatric	10–20	M < F	Stomach	Sometimes	Epi, Mix	SDHB loss (SDH mutation/ methylation)
Adult "pediatric-type"	20–60	M < F	Stomach	Sometimes	Epi, Mix	SDHB loss (SDH mutation/ methylation)
Carney-triad	20–40	M < F	Stomach	Yes	Epi, Mix	SDHB loss (SDH methylation)
Carney–Stratakis syndrome	20–40	M, F	Stomach	Yes	Epi, Mix	SDHB loss (SDH germline mutation)
Familial	>30	M, F	Stomach, small intestine	Yes	Spi, Epi, Mix	KIT, PDGFRA (germline mutation)
NF1-related	>30	M, F	Small intestine	Yes	Spi	NF1

Spi spindle, *Epi* epithelioid

mitotic activity. It is notable that two or more histological subtypes are admixed even in a single nodule of GIST. Thus, pathologists should pay attention to the intra-tumoral heterogeneity of GIST.

Among gastric GISTs, spindle cell type is more frequent than epithelioid cell type. *PDGFRA*-mutant GISTs and SDH-deficient GISTs of the stomach are usually epithelioid cell type or mixed type. Most intestinal GISTs are of spindle cell type, and occasionally associated with skenoid fibers. The epithelioid cell pattern is rare in small intestinal GIST, but, if present, is linked with malignancy [2].

KIT, also called c-kit or CD117, is positive in the vast majority (95%) of GISTs by immunohistochemistry (IHC). Immunohistochemical expression of KIT is cytoplasmic pattern in most GISTs and membranous pattern in some (Fig. 2.2). Dot-like KIT expression in Golgi area also can be seen together with cytoplasmic or membranous expression pattern. Approximately 5% of GISTs show weak or negative expression of KIT [2].

DOG1, also known as ANO1, is constantly positive in GISTs irrespective of the KIT expression level, supporting the diagnosis of GIST (Fig. 2.3) [6]. Most KIT-negative GISTs occur in the stomach, and have epithelioid cell morphology, DOG1 expression, and *PDGFRA* gene mutation [6–8]. It is notable that more than half of *PDGFRA*-mutant GISTs are immunohistochemically positive for KIT.

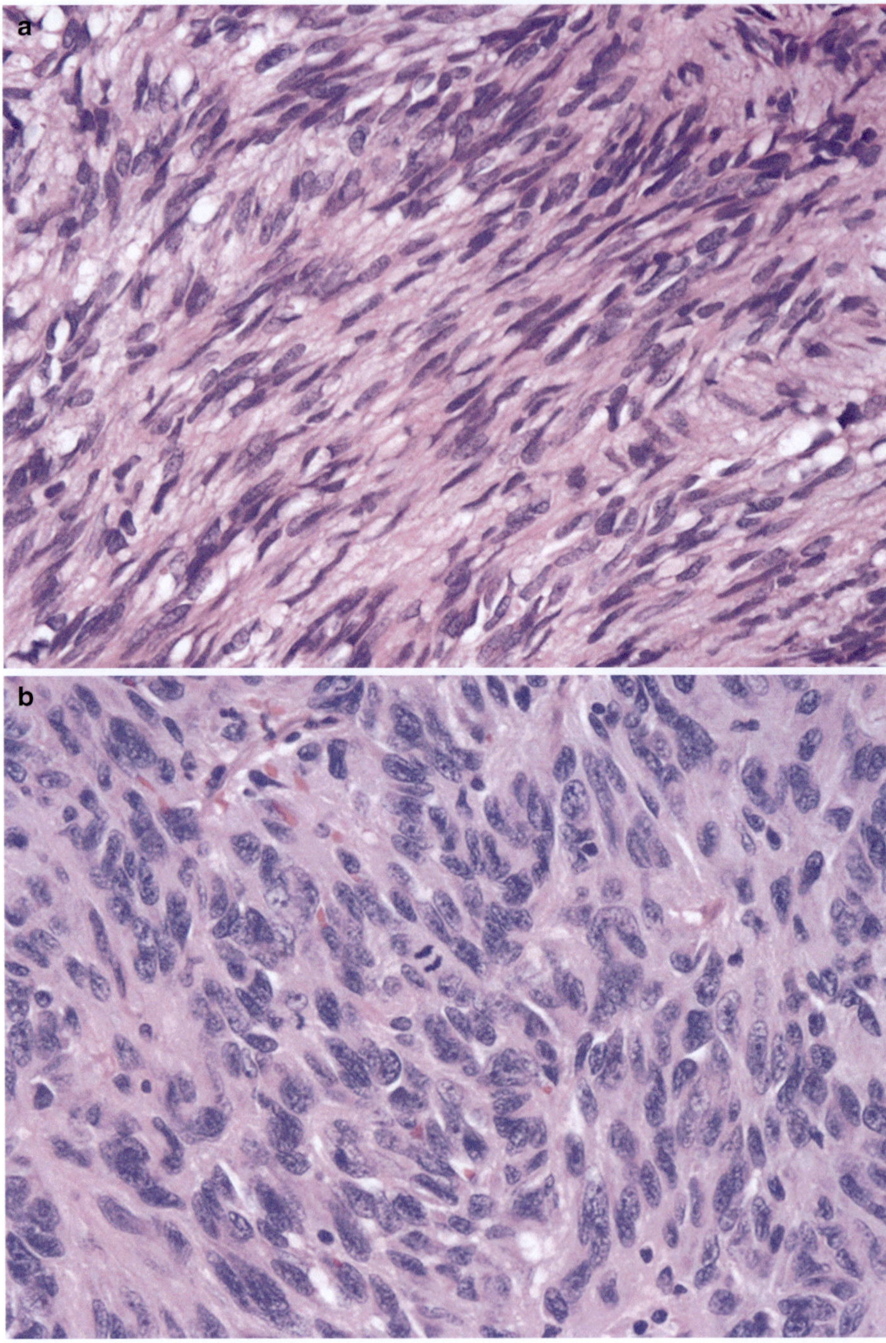

Fig. 2.1 Histological variation of spindle cell type GIST. (**a**) Typical spindle cell type GIST. (**b**) Sarcomatoid spindle cell type GIST. Mitotic figure is observed

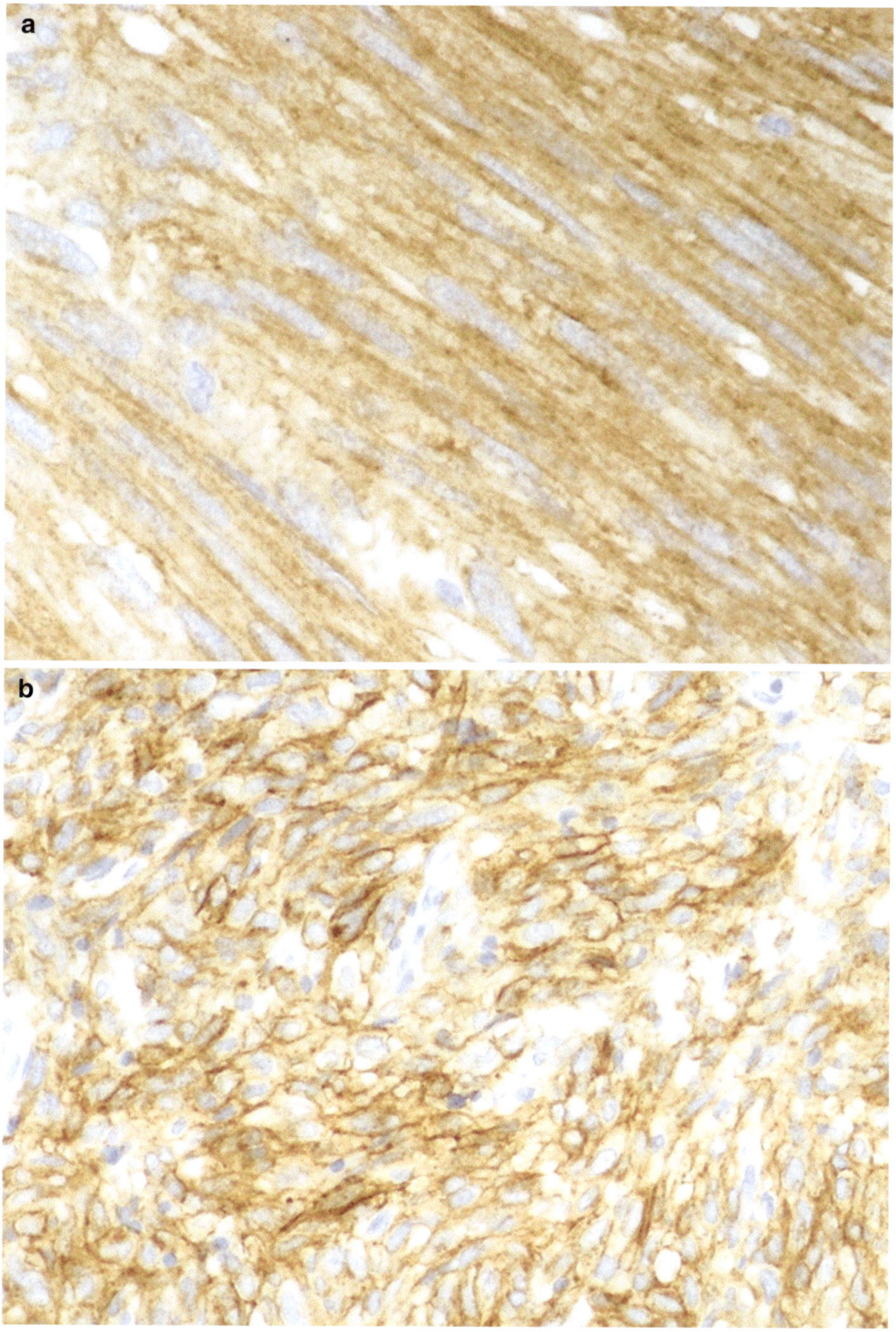

Fig. 2.2 Immunohistochemical KIT expression pattern in GIST. (**a**) Cytoplasmic expression pattern. (**b**) Membranous expression pattern

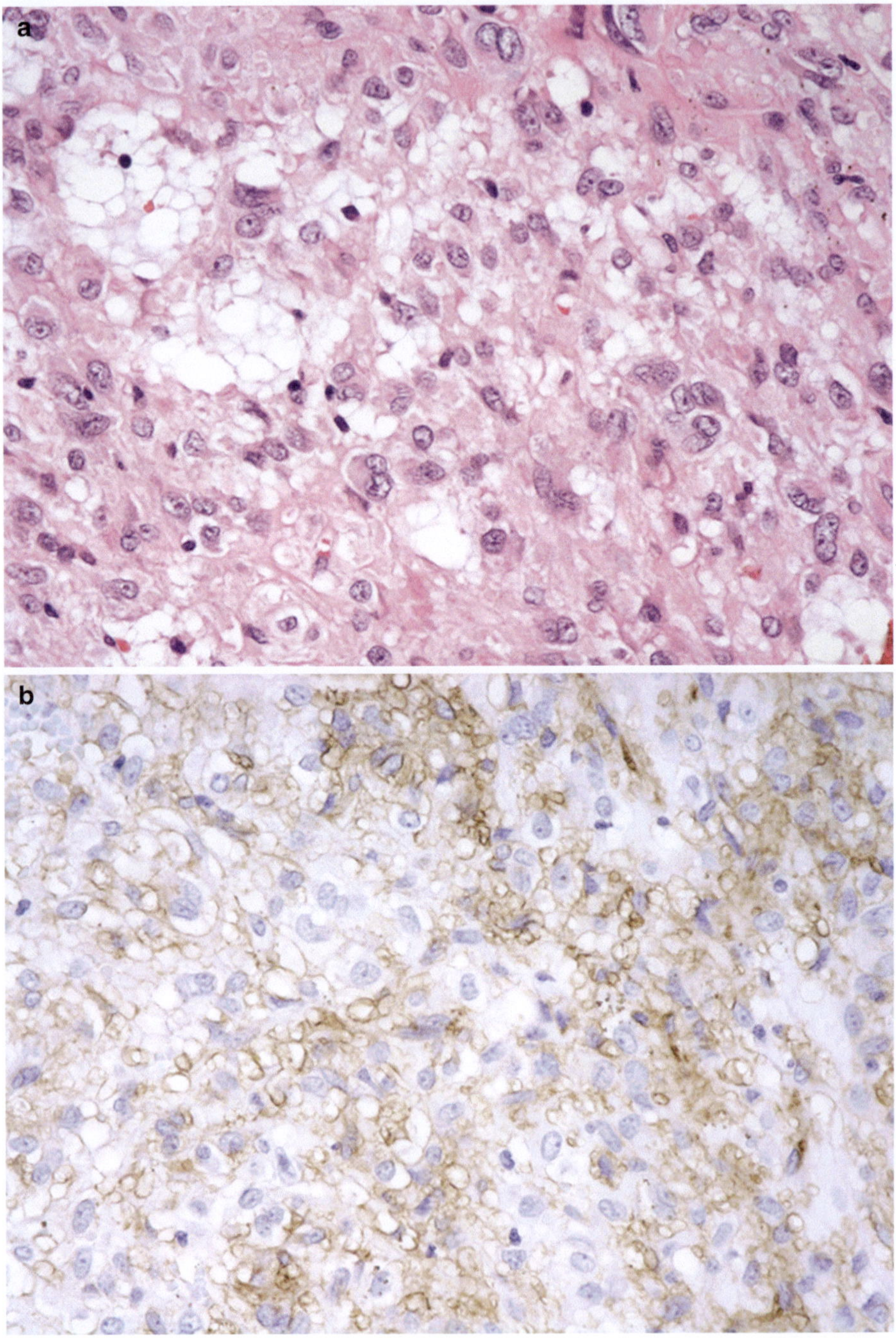

Fig. 2.3 DOG1 expression in GIST. (**a**) Epithelioid cell type GIST. This case is KIT-negative gastric GIST. (**b**) DOG1 expression

Although GISTs were included in smooth muscle tumors or neural tumors in the earlier classification, expressions of muscle marker (desmin) and neural marker (S-100 protein) are very rarely seen in GISTs. Some population (10–20%) of GISTs express alpha-smooth muscle actin. Most (~80%) GISTs show expression of h-caldesmon; however, this does not mean true smooth muscle phenotype in GISTs.

2.3 Extragastrointestinal Stromal Tumor

GIST rarely occurs outside the GI wall, such as in the omentum, mesentery, retroperitoneum, or pelvic cavity; such GISTs are called extragastrointestinal stromal tumor (EGIST) [9]. The histopathological and genetic features of EGIST are essentially the same as those of conventional GIST of the GI tract. Furthermore, KIT-negative EGIST is rarely encountered. According to the literature, KIT-negative EGIST preferentially occurred in the omentum and had epithelioid cell morphology and *PDGFRA* gene mutation, similar to gastric KIT-negative GIST [10]. The origin of EGIST is controversial. It is possible that some GISTs extend outward, losing their primary connection to their GI tract origin and eventually becoming attached to adjacent soft tissue [11]. In addition, multiple peritoneal metastatic GISTs from GI tract are sometimes misdiagnosed as primary "EGIST." However, rare cases of GIST actually occur at sites far from the GI tract, such as the omentum and mesentery, or even the liver and thoracic cavity [12, 13]. The presence of ICC-like cells in the omentum and viscera other than GI tract has been proposed as a potential origin of EGISTs, but this hypothesis should be further investigated [14].

2.4 Phenotype–Genotype Correlation in GIST

The genetic features of GIST variants are summarized in Tables 2.1 and 2.2 and also will be detailed in Chap. 3 in this book. In brief, the mutations occur either in the extracellular (*KIT* exons 8 and 9), juxtamembrane (*KIT* exon 11, *PDGFRA* exon 12), or tyrosine kinase (*KIT* exons 13 and 17, *PDGFRA* exons 14 and 18) domain [4, 7, 8]. The mutation in *KIT* exon 11 is the most frequent (60–70%) in GIST, followed by mutations in *KIT* exon 9 (5–10%) and *PDGFRA* exons 12 (2%) and 18 (8%). Mutations in *KIT* exons 8, 13, and 17 and *PDGFRA* exon 14 are very rare (~1%). Approximately 10–15% of GISTs are negative for mutations in both the *KIT* and *PDGFRA* genes.

About half of "wild-type" GISTs have inactivating mutations or epigenetic alterations in the genes coding subunits of the succinate dehydrogenase (SDH) complex [15–18]. This type of GIST shows loss of SDHB by IHC, namely SDH-deficient GIST (see below). The prevalence of SDH-deficient GIST is estimated as about 5% of all GISTs [8, 15].

A subset of remaining "wild-type" GISTs have mutations in *BRAF* (V600E), *NF1*, *HRAS*, *NRAS*, or *PIK3CA* (~1% each) [5, 8]. These mutations presumably cause the constitutive activation of KIT downstream signal pathways.

Table 2.2 Summary of phenotype–genotype correlation in GIST

Genotype	Site	Cell type	Biological behavior and clinical features
KIT exon 9	Small intestine	Spi	Aggressive behavior
KIT exon 11	Stomach, small intestine	Spi, Epi	Variable behavior Del 557, 558: aggressive
PDGFRA	Stomach, omentum	Epi, Mix	Relatively indolent Exon 18 D842V: imatinib resistant
SDH	Stomach	Epi, Mix	Relatively indolent Lymph node metastasis Imatinib resistant
NF1	Small intestine	Spi	Variable behavior Imatinib resistant

Spi spindle, *Epi* epithelioid

Importantly, the vast majority of GISTs, except for a subset (not all) of *PDGFRA*-mutants, are positive for KIT by IHC, irrespective of the genotypes.

The genotypes of GISTs are closely correlated with clinicopathological features and biological behavior as well with the sensitivity to tyrosine kinase inhibitor (TKI) (Table 2.2). For example, GISTs with the *KIT* exon 11 deletion are more aggressive than those with the *KIT* exon 11 missense mutation or 3′ internal tandem duplication. In particular, GISTs with deletions involving the codons 557 and 558 at *KIT* exon 11 are aggressive [19]. GISTs with *KIT* exon 11 mutations are usually sensitive to imatinib [20, 21]. The *KIT* exon 9 mutation characterized by duplication of codon A502-Y503 is present almost exclusively in the intestinal GISTs, and these tumors are often aggressive [7, 21]. The *PDGFRA* mutation is preferentially present in the gastric or omental GISTs, some of which are immunohistochemically KIT-negative or -weakly expressing tumors [7, 10]. Most *PDGFRA*-mutant GISTs have epithelioid cell morphology and indolent clinical course. GISTs with mutations at the tyrosine kinase domain, such as *KIT* exons 13 and 17 and *PDGFRA* exon 18 D842V, are usually resistant to imatinib [7, 21]. The SDH-deficient GISTs have distinctive clinicopathological features in terms of age (occurring in children to young adults), site (stomach), and cytomorphology (epithelioid cell) as well as frequent lymph node metastasis and resistance to imatinib [15]. Most *BRAF*-mutated GIST usually arise in the small bowel and demonstrate spindle cell morphology [8].

2.5 SDH-Deficient GIST

SDH-deficient GISTs include pediatric GIST, adult "pediatric-type" GIST, GIST in Carney-triad, and GIST in Carney–Stratakis syndrome [15, 22, 23].

The SDH complex is located in the inner mitochondrial membrane and plays roles in the electron transport chain and TCA cycle (Krebs cycle) by changing succinate to fumarate [15]. The SDH complex consists of four subunits: SDHA, SDHB, SDHC, and SDHD. Either the gene mutation or methylation in a member of the

SDH complex or an as-yet-unknown mechanism is thought to cause destabilization of the SDH complex, leading to the development of GIST [15, 18]. Germline mutations in *SDH* genes are linked to Carney–Stratakis syndrome which is an inherited predisposition to GIST and paraganglioma [15].

SDH-deficient GISTs show loss of SDHB expression by IHC (Fig. 2.4). Normally, SDHB is ubiquitously present in the cells, and thus, non-neoplastic components such as endothelial cells and vascular smooth muscle cells are always positive for SDHB with granular cytoplasmic staining pattern. SDH-deficient GIST tumor cells lack granular cytoplasmic staining pattern for SDHB. Interestingly, loss of SDHB is due to not only the mutation in the *SDHB* gene itself but also mutations in other subunits of the SDH complex [15, 16, 24]. This phenomenon is explained by the idea that mutation in a SDH subunit may cause instability and degradation of the SDH complex. Therefore, loss of SDHB expression in tumor cells represents dysfunction of the SDH complex. However, in some cases of SDHB-deficient GISTs, no distinctive genetic/epigenetic abnormalities can be found in any SDH subunits, a phenomenon for which the molecular basis remains unclear [25]. Here, it is emphasized again that SDH-deficient GIST is immunohistochemically positive for KIT.

SDH-deficient GISTs have common features, including manifestation in children to young adulthood, gastric location, multiplicity, multinodular/plexiform growth, epithelioid cell morphology, absence of *KIT/PDGFRA* mutations, and frequent lymph node metastasis (Tables 2.1 and 2.2) [15]. In addition, most patients with SDH-deficient GIST show relatively indolent clinical course [15, 22, 26]. Paradoxically, some patients live many years even after developing liver metastasis. It is difficult to predict the metastasis and prognosis in SDH-deficient GISTs by tumor size and/or mitotic counts, and thus risk grading system for conventional GISTs is not applicable for SDH-deficient GISTs [26]. Clinically, SDH-deficient GISTs are resistant to imatinib [15, 23]. Therefore, immunohistochemical staining for SDHB is helpful to identify GISTs having unique clinicopathological features and to avoid ineffective therapy.

Pediatric GISTs usually occur in the second decade with a female predominance, and the vast majority of them correspond to SDH deficient GIST [22]. Pediatric GISTs frequently show lymph node metastasis, whereas lymph node metastasis is extremely rare in the conventional adult GISTs [22].

Minor subset of adult GISTs of the stomach are similar to pediatric GISTs in terms of morphological (multinodular growth pattern of epithelioid cell), genetic (*KIT/PDGFRA*-wild and SDH-deficient), and clinicopathological (frequent lymph node metastasis and indolent clinical course) features [23, 26].

Carney-triad (CT) and Carney–Stratakis syndrome (CSS) are characterized by multiple GISTs and paragangliomas [27, 28]. CT is also associated with pulmonary chondroma. Based on the pathological and genetic similarities with SDH-deficiency, some population of pediatric GISTs and adult "pediatric-type" GISTs may be a part of CT or CSS [29].

There are some differences between CT and CSS; distinguishing features of CT include female predominance, no heritability, and absence of significant mutations

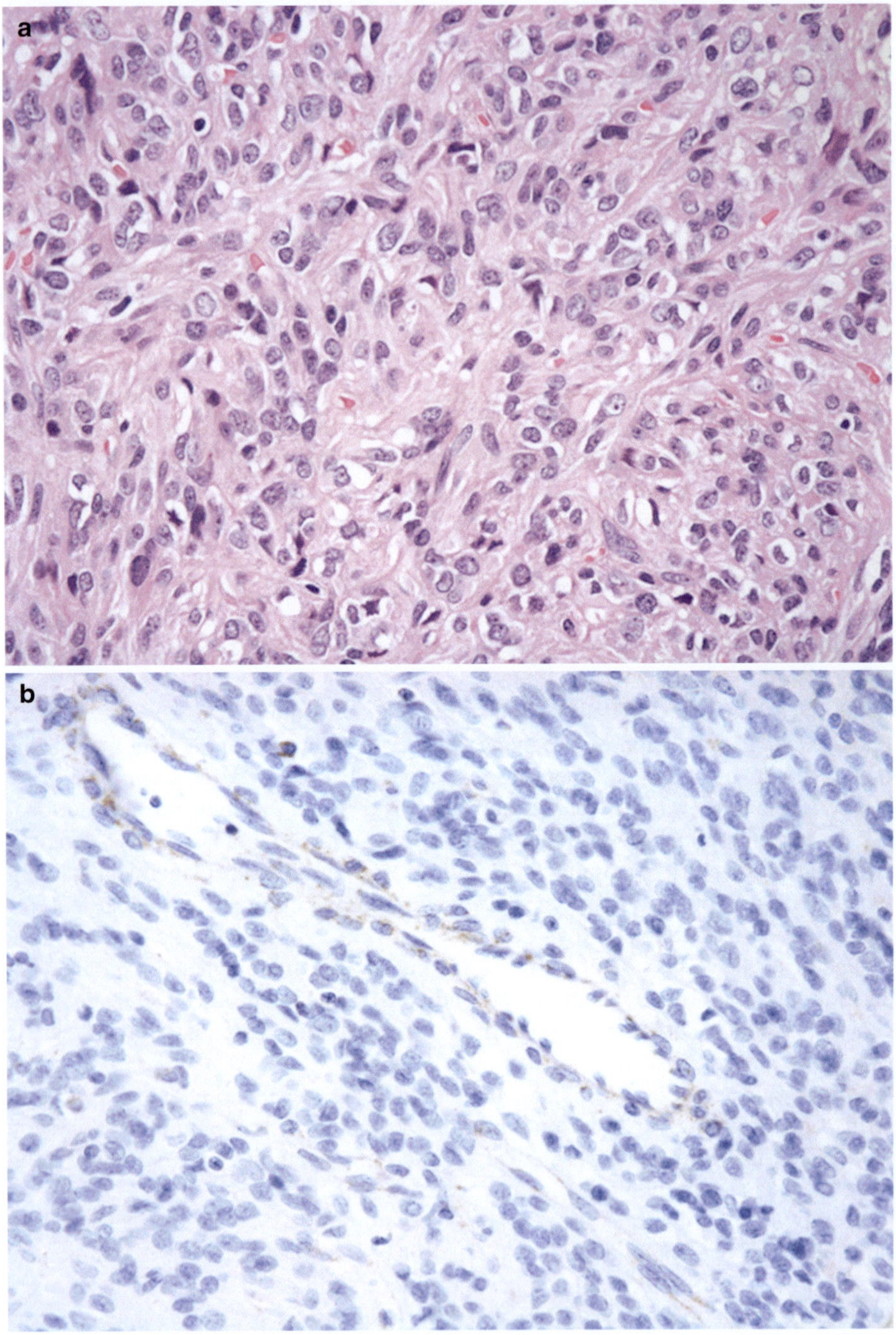

Fig. 2.4 SDH-deficient GIST. (**a**) Epithelioid cell morphology of tumor cells. (**b**) Loss of SDHB expression in tumor cells. Endothelial cells are positive for SDHB

in *SDH* genes [29]. In contrast to CT, CSS is inherited in an autosomal dominant pattern and is linked with germline mutation of the SDH subunit gene. CSS affects both males and females.

2.6 Familial GIST

Familial GIST is caused by germline mutation of the *KIT* or *PDGFRA* gene, and is inherited in an autosomal dominant manner [30]. These mutations are identical to those present in sporadic GISTs. Most patients with this syndrome develop multiple GISTs in the small intestine, colon, or stomach by middle age, but manifestation in childhood is rare, in contrast with many other inherited tumor syndromes. Some of these patients have other manifestations linked with KIT activation, including urticaria pigmentosa and hyperpigmentation. Histopathologically, familial GISTs are similar to sporadic GISTs. Broad band-like, hyperplastic lesions of ICC and microscopic-sized tumors—namely, "micro GIST" or "GIST tumorlets"—can also be found within the muscularis propria (the identical location of ICC at the Auerbach's plexus) of the same gut. The presence of these precursor lesions strongly supports the notion that ICC is the normal counterpart of GIST.

2.7 Neurofibromatosis Type 1-Related GIST

Neurofibromatosis type 1 (NF1) is characterized by cutaneous multiple neurofibromas and Café-au-lait spot. Approximately 7% of NF1 patients have GISTs [31]. NF1-related GISTs occur exclusively in the small intestine as multiple tumors with spindle cell morphology [32]. Hyperplasia of ICC is also common in patients with NF1-related GIST, similar to familial GIST. NF1-related GISTs very rarely occur in the stomach. Neither *KIT* nor *PDGFRA* gene mutations are present in NF1-related GISTs.

2.8 Quadruple Wild-Type GIST

Traditionally, the term "wild-type" GIST means the tumor lacking both *KIT* and *PDGFRA* mutations. As mentioned above, these "wild-type" GISTs include SDH-deficient tumors, *BRAF*-mutated tumors, NF1-related tumors, and tumors of as-yet-unknown molecular abnormality. Pantaleo et al. recently proposed that GISTs that lack mutations in *KIT*, *PDGFRA*, and *RAS* pathway (*BRAF, RAS, NF1*) and still retain SDH complex function (intact SDHB expression) should be designated as "quadruple wild-type" GIST [33]. A subset of this group may be GIST with *NTRK3* fusion gene. Further studies about clinicopathological, histological, and molecular characteristics and potential targeted therapy of "quadruple wild-type" GIST should be needed.

2.9 Tips for Histopathological Risk Assessment of GIST

GISTs exhibit a wide range of biological behaviors from benign to malignant. However, it is difficult to draw a sharp line between benign and malignant lesions based on histological findings alone. Based on the consensus approach developed at the National Institutes of Health (NIH) in 2001, Fletcher et al. have recommended the use of risk assessment to predict GIST behavior [3]. This risk grade was defined by a combination of tumor size and mitotic counts. Subsequently, Miettinen and Lasota proposed a grading system based on tumor size, mitotic counts, and anatomic location of GISTs [2]. More recently, risk stratification using tumor size, mitotic counts, and rupture has been proposed by Joensuu et al., because tumor rupture is strongly correlated with the risk of peritoneal metastasis [34, 35]. This modified risk classification is now widely used. The clinical significance of risk classification will be discussed in Chap. 5 in this book.

According to the author's experience, tumor rupture is often associated with hemorrhage and hemosiderin deposits (Fig. 2.5). Artificial destruction of tumor capsule (without hemorrhage and hemosiderin deposits) due to sectioning should not be confused with true rupture.

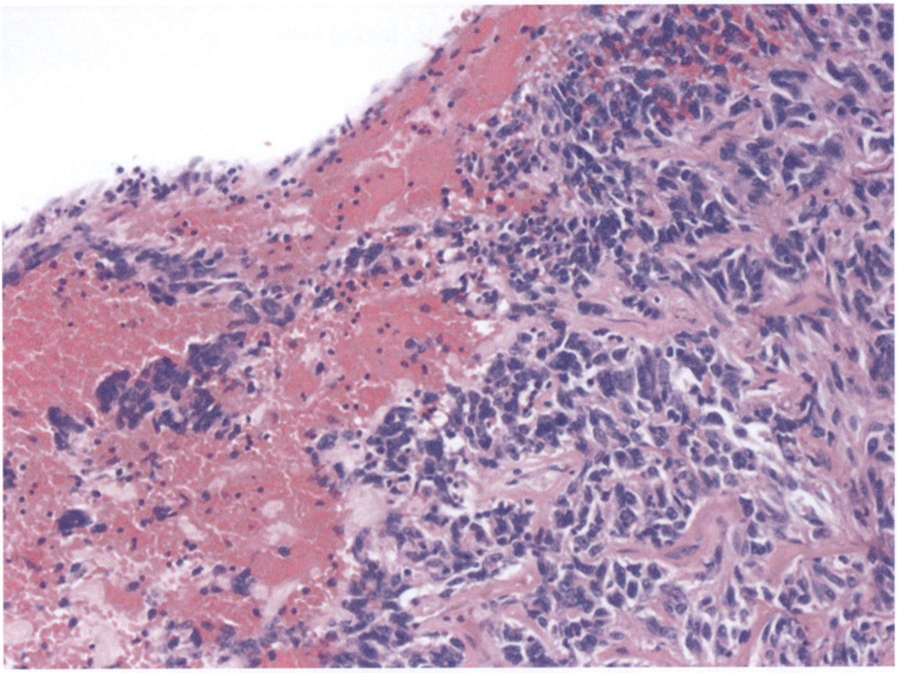

Fig. 2.5 Histological appearance of tumor rupture of GIST. Hemorrhage is associated

Pathologists should pay attention to the evaluation of mitotic counts. First, cells with apoptosis and degenerative change should not be interpreted as mitosis. If these cells were considered mitosis, the risk grade of GIST could be over-estimated. Second, microscopic field area varies depending on the microscope used for diagnosis. A recent guideline recommends that mitotic counts should be expressed as the number of mitoses on a total area of 5 mm^2 but not of 50 high-power fields (HPFs) [36].

In some cases of GISTs, mitotic counts are variable even within a single tumor. In rare instances, morphologically and/or immunohistochemically different two components are sharply separated within a single tumor [37]. In such heterogeneous or biphasic phenotypic GISTs, although the cytological appearance, immunohistochemical marker expression (KIT, CD34, etc.), and/or mitotic counts are different among the components, each component has pathological features consistent with conventional GIST. At the molecular level, each component has the same mutation (*KIT* or *PDGFRA*), suggesting clonal evolution. For the practical diagnosis, the more mitotically active component should be referenced when assigning the risk grade. The hot spot of Ki-67 immunoreactive cells may be helpful to identify the mitotically active tumor cell area.

A previous study revealed that blood vessel invasion (BVI) is a strong indicator of liver metastasis in GIST [38]. In that study, when BVI was present in the primary localized GIST, approximately 80% of cases subsequently developed liver metastasis. Among high-risk GISTs, the rate of liver metastasis was higher in the BVI-positive cases than in the BVI-negative ones (83% vs 50%), suggesting that the former can be designated as "very high-risk" GISTs. Interestingly, a small population of low- or moderate-risk GISTs had BVI in the primary tumor, and most of these BVI-positive tumors also eventually metastasized to the liver. Because the prediction of metastasis of low- to moderate/intermediate-risk GIST is difficult by risk grade alone, the evaluation of BVI might be a useful tool to predict the metastasis of low- to intermediate-risk GIST.

Dedifferentiated GIST is a high-grade sarcoma which is presumably developed through dedifferentiation and high-grade transformation of conventional GIST [39]. The dedifferentiated component is KIT negative, and is morphologically similar to undifferentiated pleomorphic sarcoma, which is quite different from that of conventional GIST. From a clinical viewpoint, dedifferentiated GIST is highly malignant and lethal, and is resistant to imatinib [39]. The details of the molecular mechanism of dedifferentiation have been unclear to date.

2.10 TKI Treatment-Related Histological Changes in GIST

Sometimes, GISTs are surgically resected after TKI therapy and serve as pathological specimens. Strict histopathological criteria for the evaluation of the effect of TKI therapy have not been established yet, and further study is needed. As for

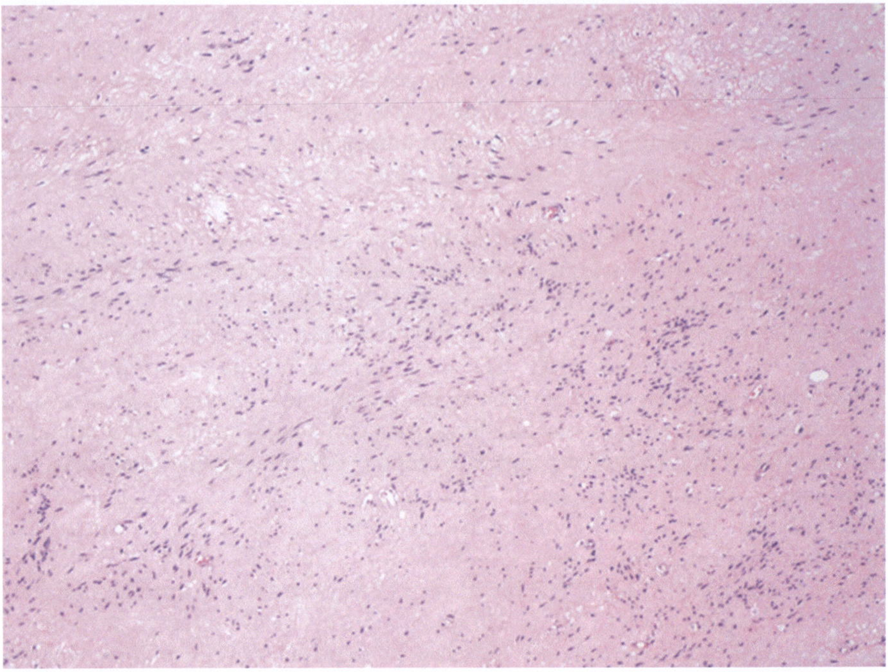

Fig. 2.6 Histological appearance of GIST resected after imatinib treatment. Spindle tumor cells are scattered in the hyalinized stroma

radiological evaluation, not only decreased tumor size but also decreased density on computed tomography indicates a response to imatinib therapy, since the latter reflects tumor necrosis or myxoid degeneration [40]. In parallel with this phenomenon, the resected GISTs responding to imatinib therapy often grossly show necrosis, cystic change, hemorrhage and extensive myxoid, and gelatinous degeneration at the cut-surface [21]. Histologically, these tumors are hypocellular with abundant myxoid matrix, hyalinization, or necrosis (Fig. 2.6). However, tumor necrosis alone is not a reliable indicator of therapeutic response, because necrosis can occur naturally in imatinib-naïve, high-grade GISTs. It is notable that, even in a tumor with good response, there are usually microscopic foci of viable tumor cells positive for KIT; in other words, histological complete loss of tumor cells is quite rare. In such a situation, assessment of the risk of recurrence or metastasis after surgical intervention is difficult. On the other hand, increased tumor size and density on computed tomography indicate resistance to therapy [21, 40, 41]. A new nodule within a pre-existing nodule represents tumor progression. GISTs resistant to imatinib show, at least focally, hypercellular proliferation of viable tumor cells often with mitotic activity.

2.11 Differential Diagnosis of GIST

2.11.1 Leiomyoma

Leiomyomas of GI tract are benign submucosal tumors which occur in the esophagus and stomach, and less frequently in the small and large intestines [42, 43]. GI-leiomyomas usually have a connection with muscularis mucosa or muscularis propria. Histologically, these leiomyomas are composed of well-developed fascicles of smooth muscle cells with spindle-shaped nuclei and bright eosinophilic cytoplasm. Cytological atypia, mitotic figures, and necrosis are usually absent, although very few mitoses (0–1/50 HPFs) are acceptable for leiomyoma. Immunohistochemically, leiomyomas are diffusely and strongly positive for smooth muscle makers such as alpha-smooth muscle actin and desmin, but negative for KIT, CD34, and DOG1. In some cases of leiomyoma of GI tract, KIT and DOG1-positive spindle cells are observed [44]. These KIT/DOG1-positive cells are considered hyperplastic ICC but not neoplastic component. Molecular pathogenesis of GI-leiomyomas has not been fully elucidated, although a previous report showed alterations in *COL4A5* and *COL4A6* genes [45].

2.11.2 Leiomyosarcoma

In the pre-GIST era, smooth muscle tumors of the GI tract were separated into leiomyoma, leiomyoblastoma, and leiomyosarcoma. The vast majority of leiomyoblastomas and leiomyosarcomas in the earlier literature now correspond to GIST. According to the most recent classification, "true" leiomyosarcoma (LMS) of the GI tract is very rare. The incidence of primary LMS of the GI tract was estimated as about 1/50–1/60 that of GIST [46]. LMSs of GI tract preferentially occur in the small intestine and large intestine, while gastric and esophageal tumors are very rare [46, 47]. LMSs of GI tract preset as a submucosal tumor which has a connection with muscularis mucosa or muscularis propria.

Histologically, LMSs of GI tract are composed of fascicles of spindle cells with eosinophilic cytoplasm, identical to LMSs of the soft tissue. Immunohistochemically, LMSs are positive for smooth muscle makers such as alpha-smooth muscle actin, desmin, muscle specific actin, calponin, and h-caldesmon. In general, expressions of two or more smooth muscle markers are essential for the diagnosis of LMS. Of note, as mentioned above, most GISTs are also positive for h-caldesmon; however, GISTs are usually negative for desmin.

Most GI-LMSs have many mitoses (>20/50 HPFs) and significant nuclear atypia as well as poor prognosis. A small subset of them show low mitotic activity (1–6/50 HPFs) and/or mild nuclear atypia [46, 47]. Even such low-grade LMSs of the GI tract have a risk of malignant behavior (local recurrence or metastasis) despite the low mitotic activity or low-grade atypia. Neither the molecular oncogenic mechanism nor an effective mode of therapy has been fully elucidated in GI-LMS.

2.11.3 Schwannoma

Schwannomas of GI tract usually occur in the stomach; esophageal, intestinal, and colorectal schwannomas are very rare [48]. GI-schwannomas present as a submucosal tumor often associated with ulceration of covering mucosa; however, the ulceration is not the sign of malignancy. Histologically, GI-schwannomas are composed of bland-spindle cells arranged in fascicular or trabecular pattern with collagenous stroma. Characteristically, there are aggregates of lymphocytes and lymphoid follicles at the periphery of tumor, namely lymphoid cuff. Of note, lymphoid cuff can be seen in minor subset of GISTs. Mitotic figures and necrosis are usually absent in schwannomas. GI-schwannomas are diffusely positive for S-100 protein, but negative for KIT, CD34, DOG1, and smooth muscle makers such as alpha-smooth muscle actin and desmin.

As for the molecular alteration, conventional schwannomas of soft tissue frequently show loss of chromosome arm 22q and inactivation of *NF2* gene, whereas loss of heterozygosity of *NF2* gene locus is not present in schwannomas of GI tract [48]. However, molecular tumorigenic mechanism of GI-schwannoma has been unclear. Interestingly, GISTs frequently show loss of heterozygosity of *NF2* gene locus and other microsatellite markers on chromosome 22q; these alterations are considered relatively early event in the development of GISTs [49].

2.11.4 Inflammatory Myofibroblastic Tumor

Inflammatory myofibroblastic tumor (IMT) is a rare spindle cell tumor that occurs mainly in the lung, GI tract, and abdominal cavity of children and young adults [50, 51]. IMT is categorized as an intermediate malignancy because this type of tumor occasionally shows local recurrence and rarely progresses into distant metastasis [51].

Histologically, IMT is composed of spindle cells with eosinophilic cytoplasm, accompanied by a prominent infiltration of inflammatory cells including lymphocytes, plasma cells, and histiocytes. The neoplastic spindle cells of IMT show myofibroblastic phenotype. Immunohistochemically, IMTs are variably positive for alpha-smooth muscle actin and calponin, but negative for KIT, CD34, DOG1, and S-100 protein.

Anaplastic lymphoma kinase (ALK) is a receptor tyrosine kinase (RTK), the gene translocation of which is present in anaplastic large cell lymphoma, IMT, and lung adenocarcinoma [52]. Approximately 50% of IMTs have ALK gene rearrangement (mostly translocation), resulting in the aberrant expression of ALK chimeric protein [50, 51]. The reported ALK fusion partners in IMT include *TPM3, TPM4, CLTC, CARS, ATIC, RANBP2, SEC31L1, PPFIBP1, DCTN1, EML4, PRKAR1A,*

LMNA, TFG, and *FN1*. Immunohistochemical expression of ALK has been considered a useful surrogate for the presence of *ALK* gene rearrangement in IMT. Recent studies reported that some population (10–20%) of ALK-negative IMTs (i.e., 5–10% of all IMTs) have the gene rearrangements of another RTK such as *ROS1* or *NTRK3* [53]. Detection of these alterations may be helpful for the diagnosis of IMT. From a clinical viewpoint, molecular-targeted therapy against ALK, ROS1, and NTRK3 could be a promising therapeutic strategy for IMT.

2.11.5 Desmoid-Type Fibromatosis

Intra-abdominal desmoid-type fibromatosis (desmoid tumor) is a locally aggressive tumor which frequently involves the small or large intestine [54].

Histologically, desmoid-type fibromatosis is composed of fibroblastic or myofibroblastic spindle cells with abundant collagen fibers. Immunohistochemically, the neoplastic spindle cells are variably positive for alpha-smooth muscle actin, but negative for KIT, CD34, DOG1, desmin, and S-100 protein. Nuclear accumulation of beta-catenin is seen in most cases of desmoid-type fibromatosis because of the presence of *CTNNB1* gene mutation [54].

It is reported that polyclonal KIT antibody at low dilution with heat-induced epitope retrieval can lead to non-specific immunostaining in endothelial cells and non-GIST tumors such as desmoid-type fibromatosis [55]. If immunoreactivity for KIT was seen in tumor cells and endothelial cells within a tumor, the result should not be directly interpreted as positive, and pathologists should consider a possibility of false positive staining for KIT.

2.11.6 Other Miscellaneous Tumors

Several types of non-GIST mesenchymal tumors rarely occur in the GI tract. These tumors include inflammatory fibroid polyp, plexiform fibromyxoma, gastroblastoma, perineurioma, synovial sarcoma, dedifferentiated liposarcoma, malignant melanoma, malignant gastrointestinal neuroectodermal tumor (clear cell sarcoma-like tumor of gastrointestinal tract), PEComa, and glomus tumor. These tumors except for malignant melanoma are usually negative for KIT by immunohistochemical staining.

References

1. Hirota S, Isozaki K, Moriyama Y, et al. Gain-of-function mutations of c-kit in human gastrointestinal stromal tumors. Science. 1998;279:577–80.
2. Miettinen M, Lasota J. Gastrointestinal stromal tumors: pathology and prognosis at different sites. Semin Diagn Pathol. 2006;23:70–83.
3. Fletcher CD, Berman JJ, Corless C, et al. Diagnosis of gastrointestinal stromal tumors: a consensus approach. Hum Pathol. 2002;33:459–65.

4. Miettinen MM, Corless CL, Debiec-Rychter M, et al. Gastrointestinal stromal tumours. In: Fletcher CDM, Bridge JA, Hogendoorn PCW, Mertens F, editors. WHO classification of tumours of soft tissue and bone. Lyon: IARC Press; 2013. p. 164–7.
5. Yamamoto H, Oda Y. Gastrointestinal stromal tumor: recent advances in pathology and genetics. Pathol Int. 2015;65:9–18.
6. Liegl B, Hornick JL, Corless CL, Fletcher CD. Monoclonal antibody DOG1.1 shows higher sensitivity than KIT in the diagnosis of gastrointestinal stromal tumors, including unusual subtypes. Am J Surg Pathol. 2009;33:437–46.
7. Lasota J, Miettinen M. KIT and PDGFRA mutations in gastrointestinal stromal tumors (GISTs). Semin Diagn Pathol. 2006;23:91–102.
8. Corless CL. Gastrointestinal stromal tumors: what do we know now? Mod Pathol. 2014;27(Suppl 1):S1–16.
9. Yamamoto H, Oda Y, Kawaguchi K, et al. c-kit and PDGFRA mutations in extragastrointestinal stromal tumor (gastrointestinal stromal tumor of the soft tissue). Am J Surg Pathol. 2004;28:479–88.
10. Yamamoto H, Kojima A, Nagata S, Tomita Y, Takahashi S, Oda Y. KIT-negative gastrointestinal stromal tumor of the abdominal soft tissue: a clinicopathologic and genetic study of 10 cases. Am J Surg Pathol. 2011;35:1287–95.
11. Miettinen M, Sobin LH, Lasota J. Gastrointestinal stromal tumors presenting as omental masses – a clinicopathologic analysis of 95 cases. Am J Surg Pathol. 2009;33:1267–75.
12. Yamamoto H, Miyamoto Y, Nishihara Y, et al. Primary gastrointestinal stromal tumor of the liver with PDGFRA gene mutation. Hum Pathol. 2010;41:605–9.
13. Long KB, Butrynski JE, Blank SD, et al. Primary extragastrointestinal stromal tumor of the pleura: report of a unique case with genetic confirmation. Am J Surg Pathol. 2010;34:907–12.
14. Sakurai S, Hishima T, Takazawa Y, et al. Gastrointestinal stromal tumors and KIT-positive mesenchymal cells in the omentum. Pathol Int. 2001;51:524–31.
15. Doyle LA, Hornick JL. Gastrointestinal stromal tumours: from KIT to succinate dehydrogenase. Histopathology. 2014;64:53–67.
16. Miettinen M, Wang ZF, Sarlomo-Rikala M, Osuch C, Rutkowski P, Lasota J. Succinate dehydrogenase-deficient GISTs: a clinicopathologic, immunohistochemical, and molecular genetic study of 66 gastric GISTs with predilection to young age. Am J Surg Pathol. 2011;35:1712–21.
17. Boikos SA, Pappo AS, Killian JK, et al. Molecular subtypes of KIT/PDGFRA wild-type gastrointestinal stromal tumors: a report from the National Institutes of Health Gastrointestinal Stromal Tumor Clinic. JAMA Oncol. 2016;2:922–8.
18. Janeway KA, Kim SY, Lodish M, et al. Defects in succinate dehydrogenase in gastrointestinal stromal tumors lacking KIT and PDGFRA mutations. Proc Natl Acad Sci U S A. 2011;108:314–8.
19. Andersson J, Bümming P, Meis-Kindblom JM, et al. Gastrointestinal stromal tumors with KIT exon 11 deletions are associated with poor prognosis. Gastroenterology. 2006;130:1573–81.
20. Heinrich MC, Corless CL, Demetri GD, et al. Kinase mutations and imatinib response in patients with metastatic gastrointestinal stromal tumor. J Clin Oncol. 2003;21:4342–9.
21. Antonescu CR. The GIST paradigm: lessons for other kinase-driven cancers. J Pathol. 2011;223:251–61.
22. Miettinen M, Lasota J, Sobin LH. Gastrointestinal stromal tumors of the stomach in children and young adults: a clinicopathologic, immunohistochemical, and molecular genetic study of 44 cases with long-term follow-up and review of the literature. Am J Surg Pathol. 2005;29:1373–81.
23. Rege TA, Wagner AJ, Corless CL, Heinrich MC, Hornick JL. "Pediatric-type" gastrointestinal stromal tumors in adults: distinctive histology predicts genotype and clinical behavior. Am J Surg Pathol. 2011;35:495–504.
24. Dwight T, Benn DE, Clarkson A, et al. Loss of SDHA expression identifies SDHA mutations in succinate dehydrogenase-deficient gastrointestinal stromal tumors. Am J Surg Pathol. 2013;37:226–33.

25. Pantaleo MA, Astolfi A, Urbini M, et al. Analysis of all subunits, SDHA, SDHB, SDHC, SDHD, of the succinate dehydrogenase complex in KIT/PDGFRA wild-type GIST. Eur J Hum Genet. 2014;22:32–9.
26. Mason EF, Hornick JL. Conventional risk stratification fails to predict progression of succinate dehydrogenase-deficient gastrointestinal stromal tumors: a clinicopathologic study of 76 cases. Am J Surg Pathol. 2016;40:1616–21.
27. Carney JA, Sheps SG, Go VL, Gordon H. The triad of gastric leiomyosarcoma, functioning extra-adrenal paraganglioma and pulmonary chondroma. N Engl J Med. 1977;296:1517–8.
28. Carney JA, Stratakis CA. Familial paraganglioma and gastric stromal sarcoma: a new syndrome distinct from the Carney triad. Am J Med Genet. 2002;108:132–9.
29. Stratakis CA, Carney JA. The triad of paragangliomas, gastric stromal tumours and pulmonary chondromas (Carney triad), and the dyad of paragangliomas and gastric stromal sarcomas (Carney-Stratakis syndrome): molecular genetics and clinical implications. J Intern Med. 2009;266:43–52.
30. Antonescu CR. Gastrointestinal stromal tumor (GIST) pathogenesis, familial GIST, and animal models. Semin Diagn Pathol. 2006;23:63–9.
31. Patil DT, Rubin BP. Gastrointestinal stromal tumor: advances in diagnosis and management. Arch Pathol Lab Med. 2011;135:1298–310.
32. Miettinen M, Fetsch JF, Sobin LH, Lasota J. Gastrointestinal stromal tumors in patients with neurofibromatosis 1: a clinicopathologic and molecular genetic study of 45 cases. Am J Surg Pathol. 2006;30:90–6.
33. Pantaleo MA, Nannini M, Corless CL, Heinrich MC. Quadruple wild-type (WT) GIST: defining the subset of GIST that lacks abnormalities of KIT, PDGFRA, SDH, or RAS signaling pathways. Cancer Med. 2015;4:101–3.
34. Joensuu H. Risk stratification of patients diagnosed with gastrointestinal stromal tumor. Hum Pathol. 2008;39:1411–9.
35. Joensuu H, Vehtari A, Riihimäki J, et al. Risk of recurrence of gastrointestinal stromal tumour after surgery: an analysis of pooled population-based cohorts. Lancet Oncol. 2012;13:265–74.
36. ESMO/European Sarcoma Network Working Group. Gastrointestinal stromal tumours: ESMO Clinical Practice Guidelines for diagnosis, treatment and follow-up. Ann Oncol. 2014;25(Suppl 3):iii21–6.
37. Agaimy A, Haller F, Gunawan B, Wünsch PH, Füzesi L. Distinct biphasic histomorphological pattern in gastrointestinal stromal tumours (GISTs) with common primary mutations but divergent molecular cytogenetic progression. Histopathology. 2009;54:295–302.
38. Yamamoto H, Kojima A, Miyasaka Y, et al. Prognostic impact of blood vessel invasion in gastrointestinal stromal tumor of the stomach. Hum Pathol. 2010;41:1422–30.
39. Antonescu CR, Romeo S, Zhang L, et al. Dedifferentiation in gastrointestinal stromal tumor to an anaplastic KIT-negative phenotype: a diagnostic pitfall: morphologic and molecular characterization of 8 cases occurring either de novo or after imatinib therapy. Am J Surg Pathol. 2013;37:385–92.
40. Choi H, Charnsangavej C, Faria SC, et al. Correlation of computed tomography and positron emission tomography in patients with metastatic gastrointestinal stromal tumor treated at a single institution with imatinib mesylate: proposal of new computed tomography response criteria. J Clin Oncol. 2007;25:1753–9.
41. Antonescu CR, Besmer P, Guo T, et al. Acquired resistance to imatinib in gastrointestinal stromal tumor occurs through secondary gene mutation. Clin Cancer Res. 2005;11:4182–90.
42. Miettinen M, Sarlomo-Rikala M, Sobin LH, Lasota J. Esophageal stromal tumors: a clinicopathologic, immunohistochemical, and molecular genetic study of 17 cases and comparison with esophageal leiomyomas and leiomyosarcomas. Am J Surg Pathol. 2000;24:211–22.
43. Miettinen M, Kopczynski J, Makhlouf HR, et al. Gastrointestinal stromal tumors, intramural leiomyomas, and leiomyosarcomas in the duodenum: a clinicopathologic, immunohistochemical, and molecular genetic study of 167 cases. Am J Surg Pathol. 2003;27:625–41.
44. Deshpande A, Nelson D, Corless CL, et al. Leiomyoma of the gastrointestinal tract with interstitial cells of Cajal: a mimic of gastrointestinal stromal tumor. Am J Surg Pathol. 2014;38:72–7.

45. Heidet L, Boye E, Cai Y, et al. Somatic deletion of the 5′ ends of both the COL4A5 and COL4A6 genes in a sporadic leiomyoma of the esophagus. Am J Pathol. 1998;152:673–8.
46. Yamamoto H, Handa M, Tobo T, et al. Clinicopathological features of primary leiomyosarcoma of the gastrointestinal tract following recognition of gastrointestinal stromal tumours. Histopathology. 2013;63:194–207.
47. Miettinen M, Sobin LH, Lasota J. True smooth muscle tumors of the small intestine: a clinicopathologic, immunohistochemical, and molecular genetic study of 25 cases. Am J Surg Pathol. 2009;33:430–6.
48. Lasota J, Wasag B, Dansonka-Mieszkowska A, et al. Evaluation of NF2 and NF1 tumor suppressor genes in distinctive gastrointestinal nerve sheath tumors traditionally diagnosed as benign schwannomas: a study of 20 cases. Lab Investig. 2003;83:1361–71.
49. Yamamoto H, Kohashi K, Tsuneyoshi M, Oda Y. Heterozygosity loss at 22q and lack of INI1 gene mutation in gastrointestinal stromal tumor. Pathobiology. 2011;78:132–9.
50. Gleason BC, Hornick JL. Inflammatory myofibroblastic tumours: where are we now? J Clin Pathol. 2008;61:428–37.
51. Coffin CM, Fletcher JA. Inflammatory myofibroblastic tumor. In: Fletcher CDM, Bridge JA, Hogendoorn PCW, Mertens F, editors. WHO classification of tumours of soft tissue and bone. Lyon: IARC Press; 2013. p. 83–4.
52. Mano H. ALKoma: a cancer subtype with a shared target. Cancer Discov. 2012;2:495–502.
53. Yamamoto H, Yoshida A, Taguchi K, et al. ALK, ROS1 and NTRK3 gene rearrangements in inflammatory myofibroblastic tumours. Histopathology. 2016;69:72–83.
54. Goldblum JR, Fletcher JA. Desmoid-type fibromatosis. In: Fletcher CDM, Bridge JA, Hogendoorn PCW, Mertens F, editors. WHO classification of tumours of soft tissue and bone. Lyon: IARC Press; 2013. p. 72–3.
55. Lucas DR, Al-Abbadi M, Tabaczka P, et al. c-Kit expression in desmoid fibromatosis. Comparative immunohistochemical evaluation of two commercial antibodies. Am J Clin Pathol. 2003;119:339–45.

Genetics

3

Tsuyoshi Takahashi

Abstract

Gastrointestinal stromal tumor (GIST) is considered to be driven by a gain-of-function mutation mainly in the *KIT* or *PDGFRA* gene. And these mutations were reported to cause ligand-independent constitutive activation of receptor tyrosine kinase, KIT and PDGFR-α, and subsequently activate common downstream signaling pathways, including ERK kinases, PI3kinase-mTOR pathways, and STATs pathways. These mutations have been reported to be related with various clinicopathological features of tumors. In addition, these findings have facilitated the development of targeted therapies with tyrosine kinase inhibitors and the revolutionary chemotherapeutic drug imatinib mesylate. Its efficacy also greatly depends on the genotype of GIST. The drug, however, met intrinsic or acquired resistance during the treatment, of which the molecular mechanisms were mostly dependent on the genotype of GIST, including primary mutations or secondary mutations in the kinase domains of the corresponding target genes, respectively. Furthermore, the efficacies of second-line and third-line therapy might correlate with the type of secondary mutations in some reports. This article focuses on the recent findings of genetics in GIST.

Keywords

KIT · *PDGFRA* · Genotyping · Neurofibromatosis I

T. Takahashi (✉)
Department of Gastroenterological Surgery, Osaka University Graduate School of Medicine, Osaka, Japan
e-mail: ttakahashi2@gesurg.med.osaka-u.ac.jp

Y. Kurokawa, Y. Komatsu (eds.), *Gastrointestinal Stromal Tumor*,
https://doi.org/10.1007/978-981-13-3206-7_3

3.1 Introduction

The major genes responsible for the onset of gastrointestinal stromal tumor (GIST) are the *c-KIT* gene, the *platelet-derived growth factor receptor (PDGFRA)* gene, the *NF-1* gene, the *SDH* gene family, and the *BRAF* gene. The effects of these genetic abnormalities are in principle mutually exclusive, and as a result GIST cases with multiple mutations are rare. It has been reported that cases in *c-KIT* gene mutation account for 80–85% of all GIST cases, while that in *PDGFRA* gene mutations account for 10%. GIST caused by other genetic abnormalities is very rare [1, 2]. In addition, recent reports have indicated that GIST cases caused by the various different genetic abnormalities have distinct clinicopathological features, including tumor site and degree of malignancy [1].

The molecular target drug imatinib mesylate, which was developed based on the etiology of GIST, is highly tolerated and has a marked clinical effectiveness, and as a result it is held up as a model of a successful molecular target drug [3, 4]. The specific genetic abnormality present is known to have an effect on the expected efficacy of this molecular target drug. Imatinib mesylate is effective on most GIST cases with the site of *c-KIT* gene mutation and some cases of GIST with that in *PDGFRA* gene mutation, but it is unlikely to be effective on cases of GIST caused by other genetic abnormalities.

Although the drug is effective on GIST cases with *c-KIT* gene mutation, in approximately 2 years' resistance develops in half of all patients [5]. Resistant GIST is caused by a secondary mutation in the gene which prevents imatinib mesylate from binding to KIT and as a result its effectiveness is lost. It is also known that the site of the secondary genetic mutation is related to the estimated efficacy of secondary molecular targeted therapy.

Elucidating the genetic abnormalities associated with GIST and using therapies that are appropriate to each unique pathophysiology are important issues for future study.

3.2 Overview of the Genes Associated with GIST

3.2.1 *c-KIT* Gene

The *c-KIT* gene has been cloned as a normal homologue of the *v-kit* cancer gene, which was isolated as the causative gene in cases of fibrosarcoma in cats. It is on the long arm of chromosome 4 (4q11-q12) and has 21 exons [6]. The encoded KIT molecule is a membrane-receptor type of tyrosine kinase protein with a molecular weight of 145 kDa. KIT has an extracellular region that is structured as 5 immunoglobulin-like repetitions and an intracellular region that has two tyrosine kinase domains: the transmembrane region and the paramembrane region. These are classified as PDGFR and type-3 receptor tyrosine kinase.

The KIT ligand is stem cell factor (SCF). When SCF binds to wild-type KIT, it forms a homodimer and specific tyrosine residues in the KIT cytoplasm undergo phosphorylation (autophosphorylation). This then activates the intracellular signal

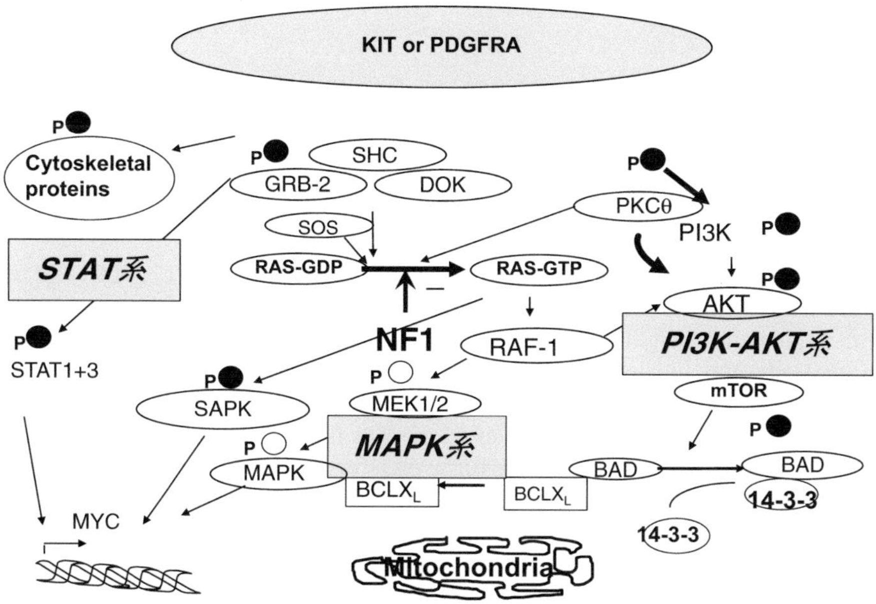

Fig. 3.1 The important signal mapping in GIST

transmission routes that are downstream of this signal, such as Ras-MAPK and PI3-Akt, which leads to cell proliferation, differentiation, and survival. In normal tissue, it carries out essential actions on structures such as erythroblasts, melanocytes, mast cells, and interstitial cells of Cajal (Fig. 3.1). In loss-of-function mutations in the *c-KIT* gene germ line, these cell sequences are deficient in mice and rats that have lost KIT function.

However, gain-of-function mutations also exist and are the cause of GIST [7]. Gain-of-function mutations have also been known to lead to mast cell tumors, some types of seminoma, and some types of melanoma, among others. In each case, the gain-of-function mutation is the cause of neoplastic transformation.

3.2.2 *PDGFRA* Gene

PDGFR, which is a receptor-type tyrosine kinase, has two sub-types: alpha and beta. The *PDGFRA* gene encodes the alpha type. It is located near the *c-KIT* gene on chromosome 4 (4q12) and has 23 exons. It has a protein structure that is very similar to that of KIT. When it binds with the same ligand, PDGFR also forms a homodimer and undergoes autophosphorylation. It acts to stimulate the proliferation and migration of fibroblasts, smooth muscle cells, and other types of mesenchymal cells and stimulates the production of extracellular matrices.

This gain-of-function mutation not only causes GIST, it is also frequently associated with gastrointestinal inflammatory fibroid polyps.

3.2.3 *NF-1* Gene

The *NF-1* gene is the causative gene of von Recklinghausen disease (NF1 disease: autosomal dominant genetic disease), which is characterized by multiple neurofibromatosis and café au lait macules. It is a common disease, occurring in 1 in 3000 people, and approximately half of the sufferers have a de novo mutation in which the disease appears in spite of the fact that neither parent carries the mutation.

The *NF-1* gene is located on the long arm of chromosome 17 (17q11.2) and has 49 exons. Neurofibomin, the product of the *NF1* gene, is an extremely large protein with a molecular weight of 250 kDa. It is expressed in a variety of tissues throughout the body, although expression is particularly high in nerve tissue. Neurofibromin functions as a GTPase activating protein (GAP) and it deactivates the Ras function of promoting the GTPase reaction in which Ras is converted from a GTP-bound active form to a GTP-bound inactive form. As a result, the functional loss of neurofibromin caused by the NF1 mutation causes the Ras-MAPK pathway, which is a downstream transmission pathway, to become constantly active. This is thought to be the cause of a variety of tumors seen in NF1 diseases, including neurofibroma. Tumors other than neurofibroma include glioma of the cranial nerves, pheochromocytoma, and GIST complication. NF1 genetic mutations are classified as deletion mutations, translocation mutations, point mutations, and insertion mutations. The gene itself is very large, and due to the fact that there are no hot spots where mutations are likely to occur and on the fact that intron mutations cause changes in splicing, it is difficult to detect this mutation.

3.2.4 SDH Gene Family

Succinate dehydrogenase (SDH) is an enzyme complex that is found in the inner mitochondrial membrane. It is a component of both the citric acid cycle and the electron transport chain. In the citric acid chain this enzyme removes hydrogen from succinate, oxidizes fumaric acid, and in return restores ubiquinone to ubiquinol.

Germline mutations in this SDH gene family have been detected in over 80% of hereditary pheochromocytoma/paraganglioma syndrome (HPPS). There are several types of HPPS. Type 1 is the result of an SDHD mutation, type 2 is the result of an SDHAF2 mutation, type 3 is the result of an SDHC mutation, type 4 is the result of an SDHB mutation, and type 5 is the result of an SDHA mutation. In general, no mutation hot spot has been identified. It has been reported that only 10–20% of sporadic pheochromocytoma cases are associated with this germline mutation. The SDH gene family germline mutation causes mutations in one allele and a somatic mutation in the other allele causes loss of SDH activity and the development of tumors. Thus, the SDH gene family is thought to function as a tumor suppressor gene. Mutations in any of the SDH gene family sub-units also are thought to be linked to the instability of and the loss of enzyme activity in SDH, which in turn causes succinic acid to build up within the cells. Excessive succinic acid buildup suppresses the function of prolyl hydroxylase (PHD), which breaks down HIF, and this in turn activates HIF in spite of hypoxia (pseudohypoxic state). This then causes promotion of the expression of VEGF, etc.

3.3 Characteristics of GIST by Genotype

3.3.1 Characteristics of GIST with a *c-KIT* Mutation

The *c-KIT* mutation is seen in 80–85% of sporadic GIST cases. Histologically, in many cases the tumor shows a spindle shape, but some present an epithelioid shape. There are no histologically characteristic features of the mutation sub-types. Mutations in the juxtamembrane domain (exon 11) are seen in 75–80% of GIST cases and mutations in the extracellular domain (exon 9) are seen in approximately 10%. Mutations in the tyrosine kinase region I (exon 13) and the tyrosine kinase region II (exon 17) are rare (Fig. 3.2a) [8].

A variety of mutations—including deletion, translocation, and duplication mutations—are seen over a wide area of exon 11 from codon 550 to codon 592 (Fig. 3.2a). This domain doesn't only interact with the activation loop to stabilize the kinase in an autoinhibited form but interacts with receptor dimerization [9]. Any type of mutation in this domain resulting in loss of its functions leads to conformational changes, to instability of the autoinhibited form, and to the loss of the inhibitory function for dimerization. Thus, various types of mutations, such as missense mutations and insertion and deletion mutations, are found in this region. There are some kinds of GIST with KIT exon 11. Tandem duplications of exon 11 are in principle limited to gastric GIST, are often found in elderly females, and have a relatively

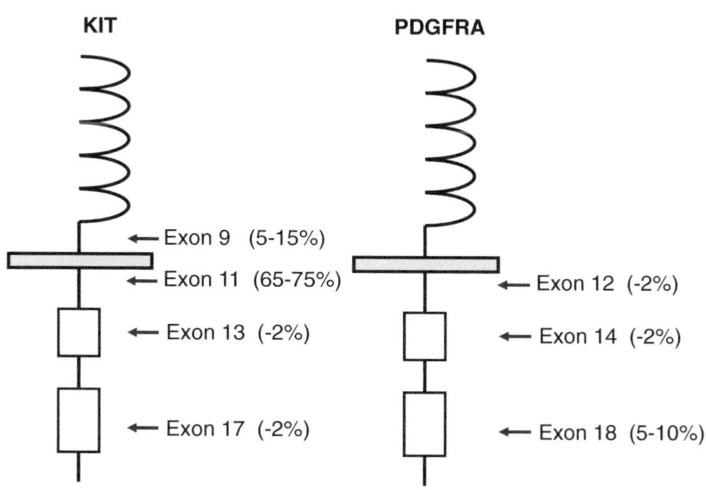

Fig. 3.2 Mutations in the KIT and PDGFRA genes. Several types of mutations found in primary GISTs and their frequency are shown

good prognosis. GIST with a point mutation of exon 11 also has a good prognosis. However, GIST with deletion mutation on this same exon 11 (particularly types that are associated with deletions of codon 557 and 558) has a poor prognosis.

Nearly all exon 9 mutations are duplication mutations of codon 502 and 503 [10]. Mutations in this region may, thus, render KIT protein prone to dimerization and this type of mutation induced to stabilize in an autoinhibited form of KIT. They are seen in cases of duodenal, small bowel, and rectal GIST (gastric GIST is an exception to this rule). These tumors show aggressive clinicopathological features [11].

Mutations in the kinase domains are uncommonly found in KIT exon 13 or 17 as well as in PDGFRA exon14 or 18. Most mutations are a missense mutation. Most of the mutations in these domains, especially in the ATP-binding domain, found in primary GISTs seem to be in an autoinhibited form under unactivated conditions, as seen in exon 9 or 11 mutations, and only the D816H/V of KIT shows strong conformational equilibrium to the activated form. In general, the kinases preferentially stabilized in the autoinhibited form under unactivated conditions are usually sensitive to both imatinib and sunitinib, while the kinases stabilized in the activated form are extremely resistant to both drugs [12].

3.3.2 GIST with *PDGFRA* Mutations

GIST with mutations of the *PDGFRA* gene accounts for approximately 10% of all GIST cases. Most occur in the stomach. Pathological examinations have revealed predominant epithelioid tumor cells in a myxoid stromal background, which sometimes express KIT protein weakly. In general, recurrence is rare and the prognosis is good. There are also mutations on exons 12, 14, and 18, which correspond to exons 11, 13, and 17 on the *c-KIT* gene (Fig. 3.2b). The most commonly seen form is a point mutation (D842V) from aspartic acid to valine on codon 842 of exon 18. And this mutation shows strong conformational equilibrium to the activated form like the D816H/V of KIT and is also resistant to both imatinib and sunitinib [12].

3.3.3 GIST with *NF1* Mutations

GIST seen in NF1 patients present mutations neither in the *c-KIT* gene nor the *PDGFRA* gene, but since most cases present strong positive results for KIT in immunostaining tests, it is easy to diagnose GIST [13]. ICC hyperplasia that is similar to that found in many GIST patients with germline *c-KIT* mutations is sporadically seen mainly in the small bowel. As mentioned above, NF1 is a functional disorder of the neurofibromin with GAP activity, and since it activates Ras downstream of the KIT and PDGFRA signal transmission pathway, imatinib, which directly suppresses upstream KIT and PDGFRA activity, is ineffective (Fig. 3.1). This suggests that treatment may be possible through the suppression of the activity of Ras itself or the downstream signal pathway activity.

Nishida et al. reported that the prevalence rate of GISTs was estimated at nearly 6% in adult NF1 patients, and NF1-GISTs may account for 1–2% of total sporadic GISTs. In addition, the clinical, pathologic, and genetic features of NF1-GISTs differ from those of sporadic GISTs, including the development of multiple small intestinal tumors, an absence of *c-KIT* and *PDGFRA* mutations, and an indolent nature. Although the NF1-GISTs are frequently accompanied with multiple tumors in the GI tract caudal to the duodenum, and R2 surgery, the overall survival rate is similar to that of the normal population with sporadic GISTs [3, 4].

3.3.4 GIST with SDH Mutations

The typical example of GIST with one germline mutation in the SDH gene family is GIST with Carney–Stratakis syndrome. Any mutation in this gene family disrupts the stability of the SDH complex. Immunostaining of SDHB is negative and enzyme activity is reduced. Carney–Stratakis syndrome is defined as concurrent GIST and paraganglioma. It is commonly found in younger individuals. There are thought to be cases of Carney–Stratakis syndrome with GIST but no paraganglioma that are difficult to detect, and it has been reported that there are cases of a single germline mutation in the SDH gene family among cases of what will be referred to below as "juvenile GIST." The relation between Carney–Stratakis syndrome and HPPS remains unclear.

Although mutations in the SDH gene family cannot be detected, as with Carney–Stratakis syndrome, cases in which SDHB immunostaining is negative and enzyme activity is reduced are known as the Carney triad, which is a rare disease that is often seen in teenage females. The Carney triad was originally defined as the simultaneous appearance of gastric GIST, pulmonary chondroma, and paraganglioma, but there are cases of incomplete Carney triad in which gastric GIST is comorbid with either pulmonary chondroma or paraganglioma. Cases of the so-called juvenile GIST, which is seen in relatively young adult patients around the age of 30 and which present mutations in neither the *c-KIT* gene nor the *PDGFRA* gene, do not satisfy the diagnostic criteria for Carney–Stratakis syndrome or the Carney triad, the SDHB immunostaining result is negative, and respiratory chain complex II enzyme activity is reduced. A search for these types of cases revealed that, as mentioned above, there are cases in which there is one germline mutation in the SDH gene family.

Thus, GIST seen in cases of Carney–Stratakis syndrome and the Carney triad as well as the "juvenile GIST" have a number of points in common: (1) No mutation in either *the c-KIT* gene, the *PDGFRA* gene, or the NF1 gene, (2) SDHB immunostaining is negative regardless of whether there is a mutation in the SDH gene family or not, (3) Respiratory chain complex II enzyme activity is lost, (4) There is a high degree of IGF1R expression, (5) Appearance is in the stomach almost without exception, (6) Often found in young females, (7) Multiple lesions commonly form in close proximity, (8) Although lymph node metastasis is common, overall the prognosis is good. The high degree of IGF1R expression is expected to be the target of therapy [14].

3.4 Familial GIST and Its Clinical Features

Familial GIST is a familial neoplastic disease with multiple GISTs throughout the stomach and small bowel caused by germline mutations in *c-KIT* or *PDGFRA* gene. After the first report by Nishida et al., over 40 families have been reported to date (Table 3.1) [15, 16]. The median age of onset (age 44 years) of familial GISTs is younger than that of sporadic GIST (60 years) without gender difference. In these patients, multiple and low-to-intermediate-risk GISTs have been seen in the small intestine, the stomach, and rarely in the colon. These tumors are sometimes accompanied by symptoms such as hyperpigmentation, urticaria pigmentosa, or dysphagia. Hyperplasia of ICC is observed histologically and, probably with additional mutation, it grows into multiple monoclonal tumors everywhere in the GIST. Clinically, it is very important not to diagnose multiple GISTs for peritoneal metastasis.

In spite of the early onset, fewer than 20% of patient with familial GIST die of the disease suggesting that most family members have low-grade risk GISTs. Furthermore, 10–20% of normal patients over the age of 60, who underwent gastrectomy due to gastric cancer, are reported to have microscopic and multiple GISTs in the upper stomach, which also harbor mutations in the *c-KIT* gene [17, 18]. Activating mutations in the *c-KIT* gene are suggested to be acquired very early in the development of most sporadic GISTs, and *c-KIT* mutations per se are thought to be of little importance in malignant transformation. These results suggest that mutations in the *c-KIT* or *PDGFRA* gene are involved in the oncogenesis and proliferation of GIST, but not in malignant changes.

3.5 The Relation Between Mutations and Molecular Target Therapy with Imatinib

Imatinib was first developed as an inhibitor of BCR-ABL tyrosine kinase and was initially used as a treatment for chronic myelocytic leukemia. Subsequently, it was elucidated that it inhibited tyrosine kinase activity by competitively inhibiting the ATP binding of KIT and PDGFR and that it inhibited downstream signal transmission. Using a theoretical therapeutic application of the drug, Joensuu et al. reported in their case report that imatinib was markedly effective in some cases when administered to progressive GIST patients [19]. Around this same time, development of imatinib as a GIST drug began. It is now held up as a successful model of a molecular target drug that has a high degree of clinical effectiveness [5, 20].

The effect of the molecular target drug imatinib on GIST is related to the region of the *c-KIT* mutation [21–23] (Table 3.2). Exon 11 mutations are in general sensitive to imatinib, but the standard dose of imatinib (400 m/day) is not sufficiently effective on exon 9 mutations. It seems to be less effective on exon 17 mutations than it is on exon 11 mutations. Although other *PDGRFRA* mutations are sensitive to imatinib, the drug is completely ineffective when used on D842V. This mutation corresponds to the D816V mutation in the *c-KIT* gene. The D816V mutation is not

Table 3.1 Familial GIST cases published in previous studies

No.	Authors	Year	Mutation			Age, years	Sex
			Gene	Exon	Protein		
1	Hartmann et al.	2005	*KIT*	8	Asp419del	60	F
2	Speight et al.	2013		9	Lys509Ile	35	M
3	Nakai et al.	2012		11	Tyr553Cys	68	F
4	Hirota et al.	2000		11	Trp557Arg	69	F
5	Robson et al.	2004		11	Trp557Arg	48	M
6	Antonescu et al.	2004		11	Trp557Arg		
7	Sekido et al.	2017		11	Trp557leu, Lys558Glu	56	F
8	Maeyama et al.	2001		11	Val559Ala	41	F
9	Beghini et al.	2001		11	Val559Ala	18	M
10	Li et al.	2005		11	Val559Ala	32	M
11	Kim et al.	2005		11	Val559Ala	38	M
12	Kang et al.	2007		11	Val559Ala	38	M
13	Kuroda et al.	2011		11	Val559Ala	25	F
14	Adela et al.	2014		11	Val559Ala		
15	Nishida et al.	1998		11	Val560del	60	F
16	Bamba et al.	2015		11	Val560del	43	F
17	Kang et al.	2007		11	Val560Gly	65	F
18	Wozniak et al.	2008		11	Glu575_Pro577 delinsHis	52	M
19	Teresa et al.	2013		11	Leu576Pro	46	M
20	Carballo et al.	2005		11	Leu576_Pro577insGlnLeu	48	F
21	Tarn et al.	2005		11	Asp579del	37	F
22	Lasota et al.	2006		11	Asp579del	58	F
23	Kleinbaum et al.	2008		11	Asp579del		
24	Jones et al.	2015		11	Asp579del	40	F
25				11	Asp579del	29	F

(continued)

Table 3.1 (continued)

No.	Authors	Year	Mutation			Age, years	Sex
			Gene	Exon	Protein		
26	Forde et al.	2016		11	Asp579del	46	F
27	Isozaki et al.	2001		13	Lys642Glu	67	F
28	Graham et al.	2007		13	Lys642Glu	57	M
29	Vilain et al.	2011		13	Lys642Glu	57	M
30	Peña-Irún et al.	2012		13	Lys642Glu		
31	Wadt et al.	2012		13	Lys642Glu	72	M
32	Bachet et al.	2013		13	Lys642Glu		
33				13	Lys642Glu		
34	Yamanoi et al.	2014		13	Lys642Tyr	57	F
35	Hirota et al.	2002		17	Asp820Tyr	71	M
36	O'Riain et al.	2005		17	Asp820Tyr	38	M
37	Veiga et al.	2010		17	Asp820Tyr	56	M
38	Thalheimer et al.	2008		17	Asn822Tyr	42	F
1	de Raedt et al.	2006	*PDGFRA*	12	Tyr555Cys		F
2	Pasini et al.	2007		12	Val561Asp	22	F
3	Carney et al.	2008		12	Val561Asp	22	F
4	Ricci et al.	2015		14	Pro653Leu	67	M
5	Chompret et al.	2004		18	Asp846Tyr	42	M

Table 3.2 The relationship between mutations and sensitivity of molecular target agencies

	Frequency	Imatinib sensitivity	Sunitinib sensitivity
KIT Exon9	5–15%	Relatively yes	Yes
KIT Exon11	65–75%	Yes	Yes
KIT Exon13	–2%	Yes	Yes
KIT Exon14	–1%	Yes	Yes
KIT Exon17	–2%	No	No
PDGFRA Exon12	–2%	Probably yes	Probably yes
PDGFRA Exon14	–2%	Probably yes	Probably yes
PDGFRA Exon18	5–10%	No (D842V)	No (D842V)

seen in GIST cases but is rather often observed in cases of mast cell tumors, but imatinib is equally ineffective on this mutation as it is on the D842V mutation. This is the reason why it is not used to treat mast cell tumors.

In the B2222 trial that was previously mentioned, the results of survival analyses conducted on three groups consisting of exon 11 mutation cases, exon 9 mutation cases, and other cases indicated that efficiency was 83.5%, 47.8%, and 0%, respectively, and that the mean duration of event-free survival was 687 days, 200 days, and 82 days, respectively [22]. The results of the previously mentioned S0022 and EORTC-ISG-AGITG trials indicated that in cases in which the 400 mg group was unresponsive, there was clinical merit in increasing the dose to 800 mg. Nearly all of the unresponsive cases in the 400 mg group were those with *c-KIT* exon 9 mutations. Thus, it is possible that it would be beneficial to utilize a dose of 800 mg in such cases. Recently, it has been determined that there are differences in the therapeutic outcomes depending upon the specific codon that is the site of the mutation, even in cases of mutations on the same exon. It is therefore possible that in the future separate treatments for each will be developed.

Adjuvant imatinib therapy has been attempted to prevent recurrence after complete removal of GIST and 3 years of adjuvant imatinib administration improved recurrence-free survival (RFS) and overall survival of GIST patients who are at a high risk of recurrence compared with 1 year of imatinib [24, 25]. The RFS was reported to be influenced by genotype. The patients with GIST with *c-KIT* gene exon 11 mutation benefited from the longer treatment, whereas no significant improvement over 12 months of imatinib was found in the subsets of patients whose GIST harbored *c-KIT* gene exon 9 mutation or *PDGFRA* gene exon 18 mutation or patients who had no mutation in these genes. Based on these results, it may become important to make a decision for adaptation for adjuvant setting using genomic testing.

3.6 Molecular Mechanisms of Resistance to Imatinib

Imatinib uptake occurs in tumor cells, where it inhibits the activity of tyrosine kinase by competitively inhibiting the ATP-binding site of KIT or PDGFRα. In cases in which the kinase is of the autoinhibited form, it binds easily and has an inhibition action, but when there is a mutation in the activation loop in the kinase region, often the activated form is almost completely unable to bind. As a result, the drug sensitivity differs depending upon the site of the genetic mutation, which in turn influences the drug's efficacy.

Half of GISTs under imatinib therapy will show resistance within 2 years. Resistance to imatinib is divided into two categories, primary resistance and secondary resistance. Primary resistance is defined as progression of the disease before any significant effects occur and secondary resistance is defined as disease progression after significant effects.

Primary resistance usually appears as enlargement of preexisting tumors or as the appearance of new lesion. Primary resistance was shown to be correlated with the genotype [26–29]. Resistance to imatinib was frequently seen in GISTs without mutations in the *c-KIT* and *PDGFRA* genes, as well as being seen in GISTs with resistant types of mutations in kinase domains (i.e., D816H/V of *c-KIT* and D842V of *PDGFRA*), and GISTs with *c-KIT* exon 9 mutations.

Secondary resistance is mainly due to secondary mutations of the *c-KIT* or *PDGFRA* gene (70–80%) (Fig. 3.3), and is partly due to the overexpression of KIT and/or an increase in the copy number of mutated KIT (10%), as well as being partly due to a gain of new but unknown proliferation mechanisms with a concomitant loss of KIT control (10%) [30, 31]. Secondary mutation in the kinase domains is accompanied by concomitant re-activation of the corresponding tyrosine kinase even in the presence of imatinib [32–34]. Secondary mutations also have hot spots, including *c-KIT* exon 13 (codon 654); exon 14 (codon 670); exon 17 of codons 809, 816, 820, 823, and 829; and *PDGFRA* exon 14 and exon 18 (Fig. 3.3) [27, 28, 30, 35] Secondary mutations in exon 13 of the *c-KIT* gene are exclusively missense mutation of V654A. Mutation of V654A decreases the binding capacity of imatinib, although the V654A mutation itself is not suggested to be a gain-of function mutation [36]. This mutation accounts for 40% of secondary mutations found.

Fig. 3.3 Secondary mutations in the *c-KIT* and *PDGFRA* genes. A representative mutations (>5%) found in secondarily resistant GISTs are shown

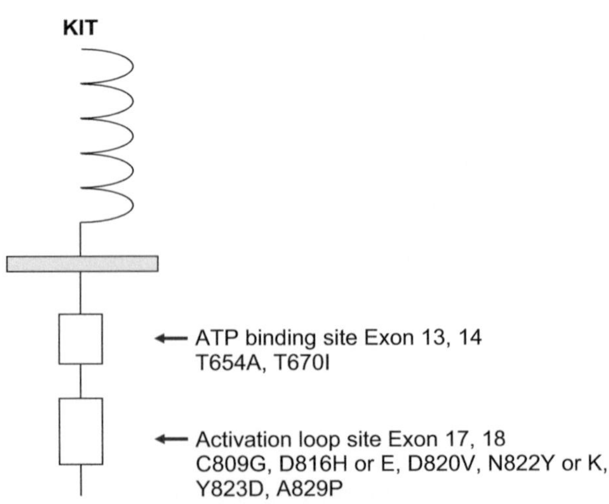

Secondary mutations found in exon 14 are mostly T670I, which is called a gatekeeper mutation, as reported in other diseases and other genes [37]. This type of mutation causes steric hindrance for imatinib binding to KIT and also induces autophosphorylation of the kinase by itself, suggesting a gain-of-function mutation [38]. In GISTs, this gatekeeper mutation was observed in 10% of secondary mutations in the KIT gene. Thus, secondary mutations in the ATP-binding domain are mostly confined to the missense mutations in two codons, V654A and T670I, which account for half of the secondary mutations in the *c-KIT* gene. KIT or PDGFRA kinase with these mutations in the ATP-binding domain is thought to be stabilized in an autoinhibited form and these forms are sensitive to sunitinib even after they become imatinib resistant [12].

In the activation loop, missense mutations were frequently detected in codons 816, 820, 822, and 823, and a few deletion mutations were reported. Some mutations found in codons D816, D820, and N822 of secondary resistant GISTs had amino acid replacements similar to those found in the primary GIST, while other mutations were novel and specific for resistant GISTs. The substituted amino acids are relatively constant, as shown in Fig. 3.3, and most of these mutations are thought to cause autophosphorylation and activation of the kinase. Some mutations found in the activation loop may be considered to destabilize the autoinhibited form by negatively influencing the inhibitory conformation of the juxtamembrane domain, resulting in a shift of conformational equilibrium toward the activated form [12].

Investigation of clinical data from the development stage of sunitinib, which is to be used in GIST cases that are intolerant of imatinib, which is analyzing subsets based on genotype, is currently under way [27, 28]. According to these analyses, the median progression-free survival results for sunitinib used on pre-imatinib samples of exon 9 mutations, wild type, and exon 11 mutations in the *c-KIT* gene were 19.4 months, 19.0 months, and 5.1 months, respectively. The clinical efficacy rates (CR/PR/SD for at least 6 months.) were 58%, 56%, and 34%, respectively. These results suggest that sunitinib is more effective on exon 9 mutations than on exon 11 mutations in cases of imatinib-resistance GIST. Furthermore, analyzing the correlation between second mutations and the efficacy of sunitinib, some reports suggested that GISTs with secondary *c-KIT* mutations in the ATP-binding domain (KIT exons 13 and 14) were sensitive to sunitinib, while GISTs with mutations in the activation loop (*c-KIT* exons 16, 17, and 18 and *PDGFRA* exon 18) were resistant to sunitinib (Fig. 3.3b) [27, 28, 30]. The correlation of genotype with sunitinib activity appeared to be true for each metastatic lesion of GIST. However, for an individual person treated with sunitinib, the genotype did not always reflect the clinical outcome of the patient, because each patient may have multiple resistant lesions which have different resistance mechanisms and different secondary mutations, resulting in differing sunitinib sensitivities.

Regorafenib was approved by the FDA in 2013 to treat advanced GISTs that cannot be surgically removed and are resistant to other TKIs, and it is considered as third-line TKI [39]. The long-term follow-up results of the multicenter phase II trial of regorafenib in patients with metastatic or unresectable GISTs after failure of imatinib and sunitinib showed benefit in patients with primary KIT exon 11 mutations and SDH-deficient GISTs [40]. In addition, regorafenib might be sensitive for GISTs with mutations in the activation loop (*c-KIT* exons 16, 17, and 18 and *PDGFRA* exon 18).

3.7 Liquid Biopsy in Gastrointestinal Stromal Tumors

To date, tumor tissue extracted from specimens obtained by surgical or biopsy procedures has been the only source of the tumor DNA required for the genomic assessment of cancer. However, tumor tissue sampling has several clinical limitations: for example, the invasiveness of these procedures precludes repeated sampling. Thus, it is possible to obtain only a static molecular picture of the disease, a picture that lacks the inter- and intra-metastatic molecular heterogeneity that characterizes most GIST.

Circulating tumor DNA (ctDNA) is a part of cell-free DNA (cfDNA) that is a small fragment of nucleic acids in the cell-free fraction of the blood, which is derived from cancer. ctDNA carries tumor-specific mutations and the levels of ctDNA correlate with tumor burden, thus it is an emerging candidate for a biomarker which reflects resistance to therapy and disease progression. Maier et al. detected the first mutations of CKIT and platelet-derived growth factor receptor α (PDGFRA) in ctDNA and showed that the fraction of ctDNA correlated with treatment response [41]. Kang et al. detected the secondary mutations in ctDNA of patients with GIST by next-generation sequencing [42], and Wada et al. showed that the secondary mutations they found in ctDNA correlated with the disease control state in one recurrent GIST case [43]. However, the application possibility of clinical practice remains unknown because of small number of patients. A large-scale prospective trial is now planning to detect the secondary mutations of imatinib-resistant GISTs in ctDNA, which contributes to the selection of targeted agents and the prediction of treatment efficacies in patients with imatinib-resistant GIST.

3.8 Conclusion

We have provided an overview of GIST as a molecularly characterized cancer (Fig. 3.4). Almost all of GISTs have gain-of-function mutations in the *c-KIT* or *PDGFRA* gene, which are targets of imatinib, sunitinib and regorafenib. Imatinib showed high efficacy, depending on genotype. The drug, however, has met with acquired resistance during treatment, of which the molecular mechanisms have been elucidated to be mostly secondary mutations in the kinase domains of the corresponding targeted genes. In addition, sunitinib and regorafenib have also encountered primary and secondary resistance, depending on the genotype of the imatinib-resistant GIST. Molecular-targeted agents should be developed based on molecular mechanisms.

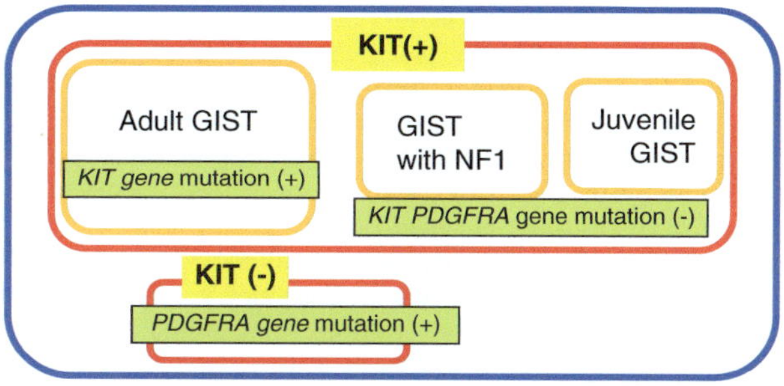

Fig. 3.4 The classification of GIST based on molecular type

References

1. Joensuu H, Rutkowski P, Nishida T, Steigen SE, Brabec P, Plank L, Nilsson B, Braconi C, Bordoni A, Magnusson MK, Sufliarsky J, Federico M, Jonasson JG, Hostein I, Bringuier PP, Emile JF. KIT and PDGFRA mutations and the risk of GI stromal tumor recurrence. J Clin Oncol. 2015;33(6):634–42.
2. Lasota J, Miettinen M. KIT and PDGFRA mutations in gastrointestinal stromal tumors (GISTs). Semin Diagn Pathol. 2006;23(2):91–102.
3. Nishida T, Tsujimoto M, Takahashi T, Hirota S, Blay JY, Wataya-Kaneda M. Gastrointestinal stromal tumors in Japanese patients with neurofibromatosis type I. J Gastroenterol. 2016;51(6):571–8.
4. Nishida T, Blay JY, Hirota S, Kitagawa Y, Kang YK. The standard diagnosis, treatment, and follow-up of gastrointestinal stromal tumors based on guidelines. Gastric Cancer. 2016;19(1):3–14.
5. Demetri GD, von Mehren M, Blanke CD, Van den Abbeele AD, Eisenberg B, Roberts PJ, Heinrich MC, Tuveson DA, Singer S, Janicek M, Fletcher JA, Silverman SG, Silberman SL, Capdeville R, Kiese B, Peng B, Dimitrijevic S, Druker BJ, Corless C, Fletcher CD, Joensuu H. Efficacy and safety of imatinib mesylate in advanced gastrointestinal stromal tumors. N Engl J Med. 2002;347(7):472–80.
6. Hirota S, Ohashi A, Nishida T, Isozaki K, Kinoshita K, Shinomura Y, Kitamura Y. Gain-of-function mutations of platelet-derived growth factor receptor alpha gene in gastrointestinal stromal tumors. Gastroenterology. 2003;125(3):660–7.
7. Hirota S, Isozaki K, Moriyama Y, Hashimoto K, Nishida T, Ishiguro S, Kawano K, Hanada M, Kurata A, Takeda M, Muhammad Tunio G, Matsuzawa Y, Kanakura Y, Shinomura Y, Kitamura Y. Gain-of-function mutations of c-kit in human gastrointestinal stromal tumors. Science. 1998;279(5350):577–80.
8. Taniguchi M, Nishida T, Hirota S, Isozaki K, Ito T, Nomura T, Matsuda H, Kitamura Y. Effect of c-kit mutation on prognosis of gastrointestinal stromal tumors. Cancer Res. 1999;59(17):4297–300.
9. Roskoski R Jr. Structure and regulation of Kit protein-tyrosine kinase – the stem cell factor receptor. Biochem Biophys Res Commun. 2005;338:1307–15.
10. Nishida T, Takahashi T, Nakajima K, Tsujinaka T, Hirota S. KIT and PDGFRA mutations of gastrointestinal stromal tumor. J Clin Oncol. 2009;27(15s (Suppl)):abstract 10560.
11. Lasota J, Miettinen M. Clinical significance of oncogenic KIT and PDGFRA mutations in gastrointestinal stromal tumours. Histopathology. 2008;53:245–66.
12. Gajiwala KS, Wu JC, Christensen J, Deshmukh GD, Diehl W, DiNitto JP, et al. KIT kinase mutants show unique mechanisms of drug resistance to imatinib and sunitinib in gastrointestinal stromal tumor patients. Proc Natl Acad Sci U S A. 2009;106:1542–7.

13. Kinoshita K, Hirota S, Isozaki K, Ohashi A, Nishida T, Kitamura Y, Shinomura Y, Matsuzawa Y. Absence of c-kit gene mutations in gastrointestinal stromal tumours from neurofibromatosis type 1 patients. J Pathol. 2004;202(1):80–5.
14. Lasota J, Wang Z, Kim SY, Helman L, Miettinen M. Expression of the receptor for type i insulin-like growth factor (IGF1R) in gastrointestinal stromal tumors: an immunohistochemical study of 1078 cases with diagnostic and therapeutic implications. Am J Surg Pathol. 2013;37(1):114–9.
15. Nishida T, Hirota S, Taniguchi M, Hashimoto K, Isozaki K, Nakamura H, Kanakura Y, Tanaka T, Takabayashi A, Matsuda H, Kitamura Y. Familial gastrointestinal stromal tumours with germline mutation of the KIT gene. Nat Genet. 1998;19:323–4.
16. Sekido Y, Ohigashi S, Takahashi T, Hayashi N, Suzuki K, Hirota S. Familial gastrointestinal stromal tumor with germline KIT mutations accompanying hereditary breast and ovarian cancer syndrome. Anticancer Res. 2017;37(3):1425–31.
17. Kawanowa K, Sakuma Y, Sakurai S, Hishima T, Iwasaki Y, Saito K, Hosoya Y, Nakajima T, Funata N. High incidence of microscopic gastrointestinal stromal tumors in the stomach. Hum Pathol. 2006;37:1527–35.
18. Agaimy A, Wünsch PH, Dirnhofer S, Bihl MP, Terracciano LM, Tornillo L. Microscopic gastrointestinal stromal tumors in esophageal and intestinal surgical resection specimens: a clinicopathologic, immunohistochemical, and molecular study of 19 lesions. Am J Surg Pathol. 2008;32:867–73.
19. Joensuu H, Roberts PJ, Sarlomo-Rikala M, Andersson LC, Tervahartiala P, Tuveson D, Silberman S, Capdeville R, Dimitrijevic S, Druker B, Demetri GD. Effect of the tyrosine kinase inhibitor STI571 in a patient with a metastatic gastrointestinal stromal tumor. N Engl J Med. 2001;344(14):1052–6.
20. Verweij J, van Oosterom A, Blay JY, Judson I, Rodenhuis S, van der Graaf W, Radford J, Le Cesne A, Hogendoorn PC, di Paola ED, Brown M, Nielsen OS. Imatinib mesylate (STI-571 Glivec, Gleevec) is an active agent for gastrointestinal stromal tumours, but does not yield responses in other soft-tissue sarcomas that are unselected for a molecular target. Results from an EORTC Soft Tissue and Bone Sarcoma Group phase II study. Eur J Cancer. 2003;39(14):2006–11.
21. Blanke CD, Rankin C, Demetri GD, Ryan CW, von Mehren M, Benjamin RS, Raymond AK, Bramwell VH, Baker LH, Maki RG, Tanaka M, Hecht JR, Heinrich MC, Fletcher CD, Crowley JJ, Borden EC. Phase III randomized, intergroup trial assessing imatinib mesylate at two dose levels in patients with unresectable or metastatic gastrointestinal stromal tumors expressing the kit receptor tyrosine kinase: S0033. J Clin Oncol. 2008;26(4):626–32.
22. Heinrich MC, Corless CL, Demetri GD, Blanke CD, von Mehren M, Joensuu H, McGreevey LS, Chen CJ, Van den Abbeele AD, Druker BJ, Kiese B, Eisenberg B, Roberts PJ, Singer S, Fletcher CD, Silberman S, Dimitrijevic S, Fletcher J. Kinase mutations and imatinib response in patients with metastatic gastrointestinal stromal tumor. J Clin Oncol. 2003;21(23):4342–9.
23. Zalcberg JR, Verweij J, Casali PG, Le Cesne A, Reichardt P, Blay JY, Schlemmer M, Van Glabbeke M, Brown M, Judson IR. Outcome of patients with advanced gastro-intestinal stromal tumours crossing over to a daily imatinib dose of 800 mg after progression on 400 mg. Eur J Cancer. 2005;41(12):1751–7.
24. Dematteo RP, Ballman KV, Antonescu CR, Maki RG, Pisters PW, Demetri GD, Blackstein ME, Blanke CD, von Mehren M, Brennan MF, Patel S, McCarter MD, Polikoff JA, Tan BR, Owzar K. Adjuvant imatinib mesylate after resection of localised, primary gastrointestinal stromal tumour: a randomised, double-blind, placebo-controlled trial. Lancet. 2009;373(9669):1097–104. https://doi.org/10.1016/S0140-6736(09)60500-6.
25. Joensuu H, Eriksson M, Sundby Hall K, Hartmann JT, Pink D, Schütte J, Ramadori G, Hohenberger P, Duyster J, Al-Batran SE, Schlemmer M, Bauer S, Wardelmann E, Sarlomo-Rikala M, Nilsson B, Sihto H, Monge OR, Bono P, Kallio R, Vehtari A, Leinonen M, Alvegård T, Reichardt P. One vs three years of adjuvant imatinib for operable gastrointestinal stromal tumor: a randomized trial. JAMA. 2012;307(12):1265–72.

26. Debiec-Rychter M, Sciot R, Le Cesne A, Schlemmer M, Hohenberger P, van Oosterom AT, Blay JY, Leyvraz S, Stul M, Casali PG, Zalcberg J, Verweij J, Van Glabbeke M, Hagemeijer A, Judson I. KIT mutations and dose selection for imatinib in patients with advanced gastrointestinal stromal tumours. Eur J Cancer. 2006;42:1093–103.
27. Heinrich MC, Owzar K, Corless CL, Hollis D, Borden EC, Fletcher CD, Ryan CW, von Mehren M, Blanke CD, Rankin C, Benjamin RS, Bramwell VH, Demetri GD, Bertagnolli MM, Fletcher JA. Correlation of kinase genotype and clinical outcome in the North American Intergroup Phase III Trial of imatinib mesylate for treatment of advanced gastrointestinal stromal tumor: CALGB 150105 Study by Cancer and Leukemia Group B and Southwest Oncology Group. J Clin Oncol. 2008;26:5360–7.
28. Heinrich MC, Maki RG, Corless CL, Antonescu CR, Harlow A, Griffith D, Town A, McKinley A, Ou WB, Fletcher JA, Fletcher CD, Huang X, Cohen DP, Baum CM, Demetri GD. Primary and secondary kinase genotypes correlate with the biological and clinical activity of sunitinib in imatinib-resistant gastrointestinal stromal tumor. J Clin Oncol. 2008;26(33):5352–9.
29. Lee JH, Kim Y, Choi JW, Kim YS. Correlation of imatinib resistance with the mutational status of KIT and PDGFRA genes in gastrointestinal stromal tumors: a meta-analysis. J Gastrointest Liver Dis. 2013;22(4):413–8.
30. Nishida T, Kanda T, Nishitani A, Takahashi T, Nakajima K, Ishikawa T, Hirota S. Secondary mutations in the kinase domain of the KIT gene are predominant in imatinib-resistant gastrointestinal stromal tumor. Cancer Sci. 2008;99:799–804.
31. Takahashi T, Serada S, Ako M, Fujimoto M, Miyazaki Y, Nakatsuka R, Ikezoe T, Yokoyama A, Taguchi T, Shimada K, Kurokawa Y, Yamasaki M, Miyata H, Nakajima K, Takiguchi S, Mori M, Doki Y, Naka T. New findings of kinase switching in gastrointestinal stromal tumor under imatinib using phosphoproteomic analysis. Int J Cancer. 2013;133(11):2737–43.
32. Guo T, Agaram NP, Wong GC, Hom G, D'Adamo D, Maki RG, Schwartz GK, Veach D, Clarkson BD, Singer S, DeMatteo RP, Besmer P, Antonescu CR. Sorafenib inhibits the imatinib-resistant KITT670I gatekeeper mutation in gastrointestinal stromal tumor. Clin Cancer Res. 2007;13(16):4874–81.
33. Heinrich MC, Corless CL, Blanke CD, Demetri GD, Joensuu H, Roberts PJ, Eisenberg BL, von Mehren M, Fletcher CD, Sandau K, McDougall K, Ou WB, Chen CJ, Fletcher JA. Molecular correlates of imatinib resistance in gastrointestinal stromal tumors. J Clin Oncol. 2006;24(29):4764–74.
34. Takahashi T, Elzawahry A, Mimaki S, Furukawa E, Nakatsuka R, Nakamura H, Nishigaki T, Serada S, Naka T, Hirota S, Shibata T, Tsuchihara K, Nishida T, Kato M. Genomic and transcriptomic analysis of imatinib resistance in gastrointestinal stromal tumors. Genes Chromosom Cancer. 2017;56(4):303–13.
35. Lim KH, Huang MJ, Chen LT, Wang TE, Liu CL, Chang CS, Liu MC, Hsieh RK, Tzen CY. Molecular analysis of secondary kinase mutations in imatinib-resistant gastrointestinal stromal tumors. Med Oncol. 2008;25(2):207–13.
36. Roberts KG, Odell AF, Byrnes EM, Baleato RM, Griffith R, Lyons AB, Ashman LK. Resistance to c-KIT kinase inhibitors conferred by V654A mutation. Mol Cancer Ther. 2007;6:1159–66.
37. Shah NP, Nicoll JM, Nagar B, Gorre ME, Paquette RL, Kuriyan J, Sawyers CL. Multiple BCR-ABL kinase domain mutations confer polyclonal resistance to the tyrosine kinase inhibitor imatinib (STI571) in chronic phase and blast crisis chronic myeloid leukemia. Cancer Cell. 2002;2:117–25.
38. Tamborini E, Pricl S, Negri T, Lagonigro MS, Miselli F, Greco A, Gronchi A, Casali PG, Ferrone M, Fermeglia M, Carbone A, Pierotti MA, Pilotti S. Functional analyses and molecular modeling of two c-Kit mutations responsible for imatinib secondary resistance in GIST patients. Oncogene. 2006;25:6140–6.
39. Demetri GD, Reichardt P, Kang YK, Blay JY, Rutkowski P, Gelderblom H, Hohenberger P, Leahy M, von Mehren M, Joensuu H, Badalamenti G, Blackstein M, Le Cesne A, Schöffski P, Maki RG, Bauer S, Nguyen BB, Xu J, Nishida T, Chung J, Kappeler C, Kuss I, Laurent D, Casali PG. Efficacy and safety of regorafenib for advanced gastrointestinal stromal tumours

after failure of imatinib and sunitinib (GRID): an international, multicentre, randomised, placebo-controlled, phase 3 trial. Lancet. 2013;381(9863):295–302.
40. Ben-Ami E, Barysauskas CM, von Mehren M, Heinrich MC, Corless CL, Butrynski JE, Morgan JA, Wagner AJ, Choy E, Yap JT, Van den Abbeele AD, Solomon SM, Fletcher JA, Demetri GD, George S. Long-term follow-up results of the multicenter phase II trial of regorafenib in patients with metastatic and/or unresectable GI stromal tumor after failure of standard tyrosine kinase inhibitor therapy. Ann Oncol. 2016;27(9):1794–9.
41. Maier J, Lange T, Kerle I, et al. Detection of mutant free circulating tumor DNA in the plasma of patients with gastrointestinal stromal tumor harboring activating mutations of CKIT or PDGFRA. Clin Cancer Res. 2013;19:4854–67.
42. Kang G, Bae BN, Sohn BS, Pyo JS, Kang GH, Kim KM. Detection of KIT and PDGFRA mutations in the plasma of patients with gastrointestinal stromal tumor. Target Oncol. 2015;10:597–601.
43. Wada N, Kurokawa Y, Takahashi T, Hamakawa T, Hirota S, Naka T, Miyazaki Y, Makino T, Yamasaki M, Nakajima K, Takiguchi S, Mori M, Doki Y. Detecting secondary C-KIT mutations in the peripheral blood of patients with imatinib-resistant gastrointestinal stromal tumor. Oncology. 2016;90(2):112–7. https://doi.org/10.1159/000442948.

Diagnostic Imaging of Gastrointestinal Stromal Tumor

4

Tomohiro Yoneyama, Bae Hyeyeol, Yoshio Kitazume, Mitsuhiro Kishino, and Ukihide Tateishi

Abstract

GIST is the most frequent mesenchymal tumor in the digestive tract. Imaging modalities comprising of ultrasound, computed tomography (CT), magnetic resonance imaging (MRI), and positron emission tomography/computed tomography (PET/CT) are routinely used for management of tumor. We focus on diagnosis of staging, recurrence, and monitoring.

Keywords

GIST · Imaging · CT · MRI · PET/CT

4.1 Introduction

In 1983, Mazur and Clark defined the gastrointestinal stromal tumor (GIST) as a characteristic subgroup of gastrointestinal mesenchymal tumors unclassified as deriving from neural or smooth muscle [1]. Kindblom et al. hypothesized that these tumors may arise from Kahal's stromal cells in the normal intestinal plexus [2]. This hypothesis was confirmed by Hirota et al. in 2000 [3]. Nowadays, based on pathological features, GIST is defined as a mesenchymal tumor of the gastrointestinal tract that expresses positive for KIT (CDl17), the c-kit receptor tyrosine kinase.

T. Yoneyama · B. Hyeyeol · Y. Kitazume · M. Kishino · U. Tateishi (✉)
Department of Diagnostic Radiology, Tokyo Medical and Dental University, Tokyo, Japan
e-mail: ttisdrnm@tmd.ac.jp

Y. Kurokawa, Y. Komatsu (eds.), *Gastrointestinal Stromal Tumor*,
https://doi.org/10.1007/978-981-13-3206-7_4

GIST is the most frequent mesenchymal tumor in the digestive tract. Despite accounting for only about 3% of all malignant tumors of the stomach, GIST is the most frequent in malignant tumors of small bowel and accounts for 20%. It occurs in the stomach (60–70%), small intestine (20–25%), rectum, esophagus, colon, and appendix.

Approximately 95% of GIST is positive for KIT. The mutation of KIT leads to activation with the receptor dimerization independent of the ligand of KIT tyrosine kinase. These mutations are confirmed in more than 80% of GIST, and most of the mutations occur in the vicinity of the membrane encoded by exon 11. Mutations may also occur at exons 9, 13, 17 or platelet-derived growth factor receptor (PDGFR). At a response rate of 85%, they show significant clinical response to imatinib therapy. Sunitinib therapy is the second molecular-target therapy, which is a multi-target tyrosine kinase inhibitor of KIT and PDGFR.

Most of GISTs can be diagnosed on KIT immunoreactivity. However, some neoplasms show weak or negative KIT expression [4]. They are very rare, accounting for less than 5% of all GISTs [5] and usually occur in the stomach, omentum, or mesentery. The cytogenetic analysis revealed the existence of mutations of the platelet-derived growth factor receptor α (PDGFRA) gene which was also the product of the c-kit proto-oncogene in KIT-weak or KIT-negative GISTs [6].

4.2 Staging

Staging of GIST differs between gastric GIST and small intestinal GIST. In stage I–III, both gastric GIST and small intestinal GIST are classified in accordance with the size of tumor and mitotic rate (histologic grade).

4.2.1 Staging of Gastric GIST

Stage I is divided into stage I,A and stage I,B, depending on the size of tumor in the greatest dimension under the condition of mitotic rate 5/50 per high-power field (HPF) or less. Stage I,A: the size of tumor is not more than 5 cm. Stage I,B: the size of tumor is more than 5 cm but not more than 10 cm. In stage II, the size of tumor in greatest dimension is more than 10 cm under the condition of mitotic rate 5/50 per HPF or less, or the size of tumor is not more than 5 cm under the condition of mitotic rate >5/50 HPF. Stage III is divided into stage III,A and stage III,B depending on the size of tumor in the greatest dimension under the condition of mitotic rate >5/50 HPF. Stage III,A: the size of tumor is more than 5 cm but not more than 10 cm. Stage III,B: the size of tumor is more than 10 cm. In stage IV, gastric GIST has at least one lymph node metastasis and/or distant metastasis regardless of the size of tumor and mitotic rate.

4.2.2 Staging of Small Intestinal GIST

In stage I, the size of tumor in greatest dimension is not more than 5 cm under the condition of mitotic rate 5/50 per HPF or less. In stage II, the size of tumor in greatest dimension is more than 5 cm but not more than 10 cm under the same condition. Stage III is divided into stage III,A and stage III,B, depending on the size of tumor in greatest dimension and mitotic rate. Stage III,A: the size of tumor is more than 10 cm under the condition of mitotic rate 5/50 per HPF or less. Stage III,B: the size of tumor is more than 2 cm but not more than 10 cm under the condition of mitotic rate >5/50 HPF. In stage IV, small intestinal GIST has at least one lymph node metastasis and/or distant metastasis regardless of the size of tumor and mitotic rate.

4.3 Primary Tumor

Computed tomography (CT) and magnetic resonance imaging (MRI) are well-accepted methods for diagnosis and staging of GISTs [7–11].

4.3.1 CT

CT allows precise assessment of tumor morphology, composition, location, and extent. Relevant anatomy is well visualized on axial, coronal, and sagittal images as well as any oblique planes provided by multiplanar reconstruction or reformatting. CT features of GIST show various findings depending on the size and aggressiveness of the tumor [12, 13]. On unenhanced CT, GISTs typically show isodense to normal muscle, and enhancing masses on contrast-enhanced CT (Fig. 4.1). Heterogeneous enhancements are often observed because of necrosis, hemorrhage, or cystic degeneration [7–11]. Intralesional calcifications are sometimes confirmed as clinicopathologic feature of GISTs and CT is superior to MRI in detecting them. The calcifications within GISTs distribute circumscribed and patchy. They are thought to be caused by previous bleeding or tumor necrosis with cystic degeneration [8]. Time density curve of contrast-enhanced CT demonstrates optimal timing of scan delay (Fig. 4.2). Dynamic contrast-enhanced CT images provides information of tumor vascularity and blood flow; i.e., k1–k4 and areas under the curve (AUC), being calculated by two- or three-compartment model.

GISTs usually oppress and displace adjacent structures, and the direct invasion is sometimes observed with advanced disease. In the case of large GIST, the origin is difficult to be identified due to its prominent extraluminal location. Small GISTs usually show endoluminal and polypoid appearance, and are homogenous.

Tateishi et al. reported that the CT findings, including lesion larger than 11.1 cm, irregular surface, unclear boundary, presence of invasion, heterogeneous enhancement, hepatic metastasis, and peritoneal dissemination, were more

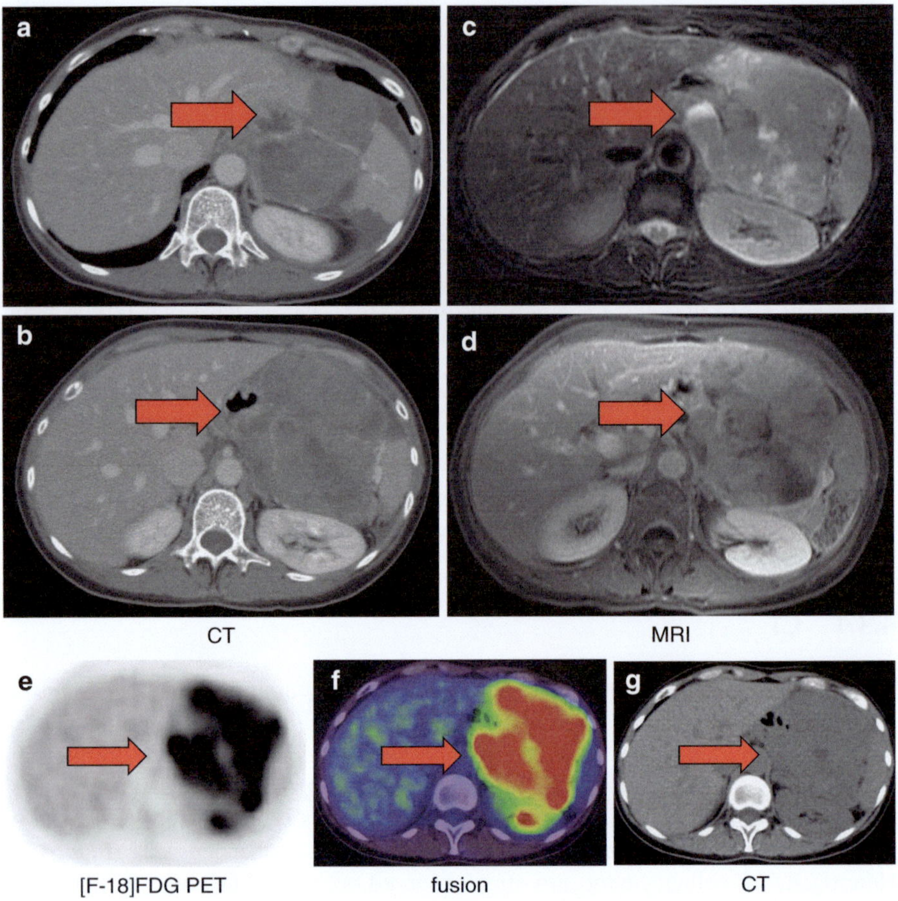

Fig. 4.1 A man of 50 years with gastric GIST. Tumor greater than 11 cm in the long axis demonstrates heterogeneous enhancement on axial contrast-enhanced CT (**a**, **b**: arrow). Axial T2-weighted MR image shows heterogeneous hypersignal intensity relative to muscle (**c**, arrow). Tumor shows heterogeneous enhancement on gadolinium-enhanced T1-weighted MR image (**d**, arrow). [F-18] FDG PET/CT reveals high avidity of tumor (**e**–**g**, arrow)

often found in high-grade GISTs and were associated significantly with decreased survival. Especially, a lesion larger than 11.1 cm, wall invasion of the target organ, and hepatic metastasis identified on CT images had a significant effect on prognosis [14].

4.3.2 MRI

MRI allows tissue characterization, accurate assessment of tumor extent, differentiation from structures, information of blood flow, diffusion capacity,

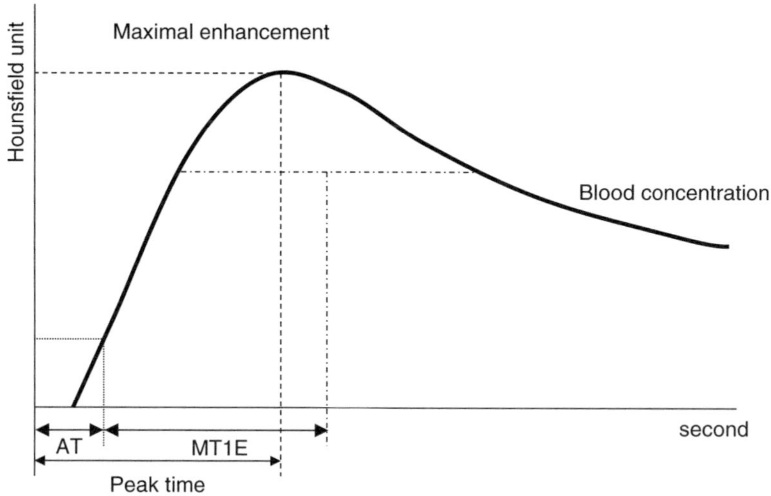

Fig. 4.2 Time density curve after administration of contrast media on CT. The curve shows maximal density at peak time after intravenous administration of contrast media. After delayed phase, tumor density decreases to blood concentration. *AT* appearance time of contrast media, *MT1E* mean transit time of enhancement

texture features, and specification of metabolites within tumors. On unenhanced MRI, GISTs appear as isointense to normal muscle on T1-weighted images and hyperintense on T2-weighted images, and moderately or mildly enhanced. Reflecting intralesional necrosis or hemorrhage, a heterogeneous pattern of enhancement is more common on contrast-enhanced MRI, similar to CT (Fig. 4.1). Following MRI findings must be collected for differentiation of tumor: tumor size, location, types of margin and contours, internal architecture, tumor capsule, signal characteristics, and heterogeneity. On gadolinium contrast-enhanced studies, the extent (none/weak or pronounced), pattern (punctate or diffuse), and homogeneity after administration are also recorded for assessment. However, gadolinium enhancement pattern of GIST is similar to those of contrast-enhanced CT.

Yu et al. reported that the features of small GISTs were round shape with a homogeneous enhancement pattern, and large GISTs had a lobulated shape, heterogeneous enhancement pattern, and intratumoral cystic change [15]. They also found that the prevalence of intratumoral cystic change was significantly higher in the moderate to high risk group than in the very low to low risk group, and the intratumoral cystic change seen on MR images correlated with tumor necrosis, hemorrhage at pathologic examination. Atypical GIST with KIT-weak or KIT-negative often showed a large extraluminal mass with heterogeneous lesion containing cystic regions and soft tissue elements in CT and MRI images. However, it is impossible to diagnose atypical GISTs from conventional GISTs, because these findings are not specific [16].

4.3.3 Positron Emission Tomography/Computed Tomography (PET/CT)

Functional imaging methods, especially [F-18] fluorodeoxyglucose—positron emission tomography/computed tomography ([F-18] FDG -PET/CT), had played a pivotal role in the management of GIST, which can provide the information of metabolic activity in addition to morphologic features (Fig. 4.1). The uptake of GIST exhibits various patterns and intensity in PET/CT with [F-18] FDG. Malignant cells are frequently associated with increased metabolic activity. [F-18] FDG, which accumulates in proportion to the glucose metabolism, is the PET tracer most commonly used in oncology. [F-18] FDG uptake is generally higher in malignant lesions than benign ones, while it is also seen in inflammatory changes or fractures. Miyake et al. classified the uptake pattern of GIST into four patterns ("Ring-shaped" was defined as round or semi-round uptake with an apparent central uptake defect, "Homogeneous/diffuse" was defined as fairly uniform uptake covering almost the entire tumor, "Heterogeneous/partial" was defined as inhomogeneous or deficient uptake, and other than above is "unclassified") and scored the uptake intensity on a four-point scale ("faint-to-none" for uptake less than background hepatic uptake, "mild" for uptake similar to liver uptake, "moderate" for uptake moderately greater than hepatic uptake, and "intense" for intense uptake equal to or greater than brain uptake). Then, they investigated the correlation between the uptake pattern or uptake intensity and recurrence-free survival (RFS). As a result, ring-shaped uptake was significantly associated with lower RFS compared to those with the other uptake patterns. Intense uptake also had a significant association with lower RFS [17]. Recently, PET/MRI has been introduced and used in the assessment of malignancies including GIST. [F-18] FDG PET/MRI possesses highly diagnostic performance. MRI also provides the reduction of radiation exposure, especially pivotal in younger patients. However, PET/MRI has the disadvantages of longer examination times, the difficulty in evaluating lung lesions and metallic artifacts.

4.4 Metastases

The most common metastatic site is liver, detected in 70% of patients followed by the peritoneum, whereas, bone, lung, and lymph nodes are low frequency as a site of metastasis [13, 18]. Liver metastases show various appearances that resemble primary lesions. On CT images, they are often multiple and appear low density mass with peripheral enhancement reflecting necrosis at the center and peripheral solid component. Enhancement pattern on CT depends on scan delay after intravenous administration of contrast agent. When we stratify by hepatic metastasis of GIST, hepatic blood flow affects flow-through pattern of contrast medium. Patterns of contrast enhancement depend on flow-through pattern (Figs. 4.3 and 4.4). Therefore, optimal timing has to be determined in order to detect more precisely based on time density curve (Fig. 4.2). Metastasis sometimes shows the variegated appearance due to protein material, bleeding, and calcification [19]. Although

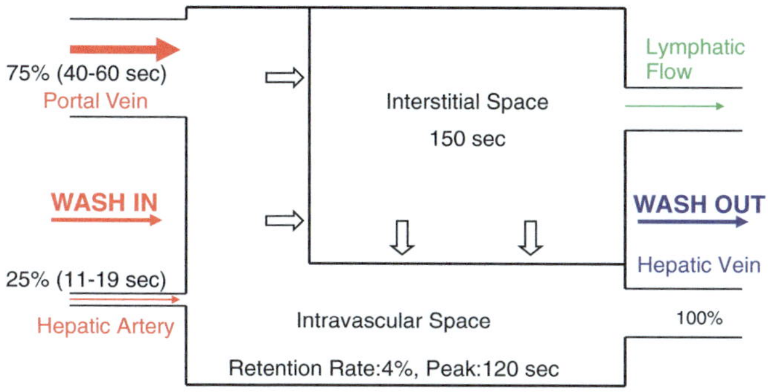

Fig. 4.3 Schematic compartmental model of contrast medium flow-through pattern. Hepatic in-flow consists of portal vein and hepatic artery as wash-in. Administered contrast media reaches to liver mostly via portal vein at 40–60 s. Contrast media doesn't retain intravascular space and move to interstitial space at 150 s. Finally, out-flow consists of hepatic vein and lymphatic vessels as wash-out

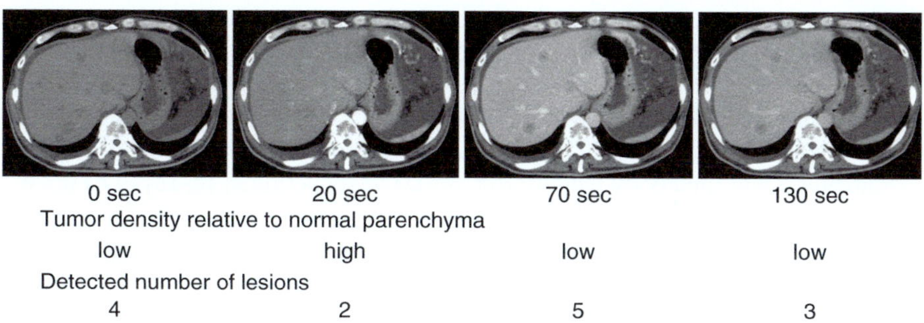

Fig. 4.4 Dynamic contrast-enhanced CT series in a man of 60 years with hepatic metastases of GIST. Visual assessment of tumor density relative to normal parenchyma and the numbers of detected hepatic metastases are presented. Image obtained at 70 s reveals maximal number of lesions compared to other phases. Optimal CT timing is important to assess hepatic metastasis of GIST on dynamic contrast-enhanced CT

gadolinium enhancement pattern of GIST is similar to those of contrast-enhanced CT, MRI using super paramagnetic iron oxide (SPIO) provides us to visualize metastatic liver tumor. SPIO is usually distributed in blood and Kupffer cell after intravenous administration. Hepatic metastasis is hypersignal relative to adjacent normal liver tissue on T2-weighted MR images. Hepatocyte specific contrast agent has been used for differentiation from hepatocellular carcinoma. Peritoneal lesions often show large discrete masses that appear similar to the primary tumor. Most of the peritoneal spread is caused by the tumor seedling during surgery and biopsy [20].

The lymph node metastases of GIST patients are believed to be 1–4% [21, 22]. However, pediatric and young adult patients have higher frequency. Agaimy and Peter reported that the lymph node metastases were observed in approximately 20% of patients ≦40 years. In addition, the frequency of lymph node metastasis varies depending on the primary site [23]. Gong et al. reported that the most notable factor of the lymph node metastasis is the location of the primary tumor. Out of five adult patients, four patients' primary tumors were located at very uncommon places as prostate, duodenum, right ovary, and esophagus, only one is in stomach [24].

Gayed et al. compared the performance (true-positive, true-negative, false-positive, and false-negative findings) of [F-18] FDG PET and CT on the pretherapy scans. The sensitivity and positive predictive values were 93% and 100%, respectively, for CT and 86% and 98%, respectively, for [F-18] FDG PET. There was no statistical difference between CT and [F-18] FDG PET in the sensitivity or positive predictive values [25].

4.5 Monitoring Tumor Response

Conventional methods to monitor treatment response are based on the size reduction on CT. However, the changes of tumor metabolism often occur early during therapy and precede size reduction of the tumor. The quantification of tumor glucose metabolism is highly accurate for monitoring effects of chemotherapy. Choi et al. reported criteria based on contrast-enhanced CT with special reference to [F-18] FDG PET [26]. They suggested cutoff of tumor response with 10% change of maximal perpendicular diameter or 15% change of CT. However, change of CT density depends on scan delay, concentration of contrast media, bolus of contrast media, blood flow, and body weight (Fig. 4.5). The reduction of [F-18] FDG uptake

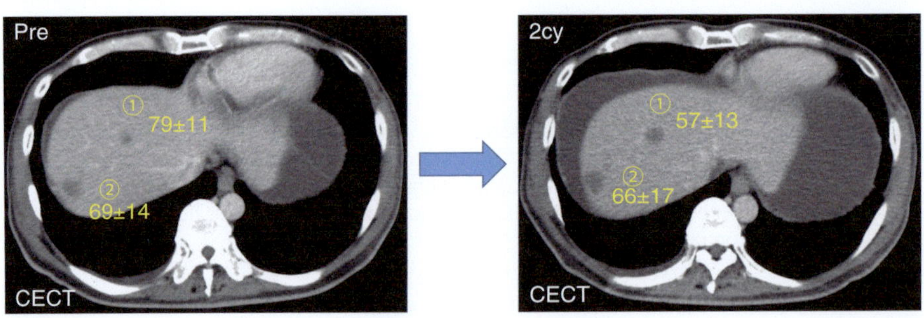

	ΔHU		
①	22	28%↓	PR
②	3	4%↓	SD

Fig. 4.5 Response assessment of two hepatic metastases on contrast-enhanced CT. One hepatic metastasis (①) shows 28% decrease of Hounsfield unit after 2 cycles of imatinib therapy and this lesion indicates partial response on Choi's criteria. In contrast, the other hepatic metastasis (②) demonstrates only 4% decrease of Hounsfield unit after 2 cycles of imatinib therapy with stable disease. Response assessment only by change of density has possibility to lead to inaccurate conclusion. General evaluation is needed for accurate response assessment. *Pre* baseline, *2cy* after 2 cycles, *ΔHU* change of Hounsfield unit, *PR* partial response, *SD* stable disease

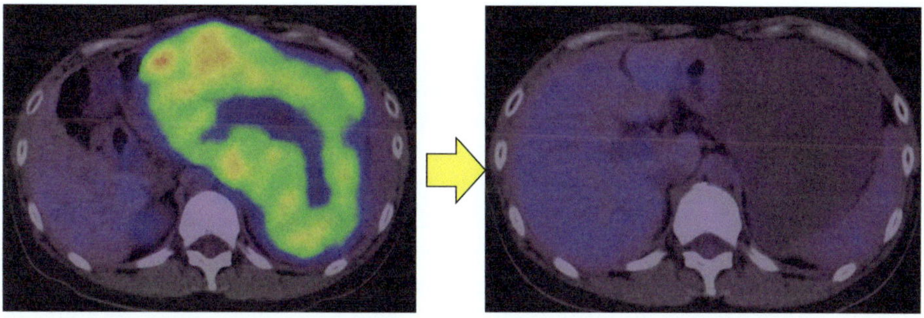

	Day 0	Day 60
SUVmax, g/ml	11.3	1.9
TLG, g	6808	440
Size, mm	144.6	88.7
Volume, cm³	1565	484

Fig. 4.6 Monitoring of response of gastric GIST. Typical responder shows parallel decrease in SUV, TLG, size, and volume during the course of disease. Metabolic response by [F-18] FDG PET/CT usually precedes morphometric changes of CT. *SUV* standardized uptake value, *TLG* total lesion glycolysis

between pre- and post-chemotherapy has a relationship with histological change, often prior to morphologic changes on conventional imaging (Fig. 4.6). Fuster et al. evaluated the role of [F-18] FDG PET in assessing 21 patients with locally advanced and/or metastatic GIST refractory to high-dose imatinib treated with doxorubicin. Of 21 patients, 6 patients had partial response by [F-18] FDG PET obtained after 2 months of treatment, 9 showed stable disease, and 6 showed progression of disease based on European Organization for Research and Treatment of Cancer (EORTC) criteria. There was a significant correlation between PET response and progression-free survival (PFS) [27].

Prior et al. assessed tumor metabolism with [F 18] FDG PET before and after the first 4 weeks of sunitinib therapy in 23 patients who received 1–12 cycles of sunitinib therapy (4 weeks of 50 mg/day, 2 weeks off). They evaluated treatment response with the percent change in maximal standardized uptake values (SUV). Using −25% and +25% thresholds for SUV variations from baseline, early [F-18] FDG PET response was stratified in partial response (PR), stable disease (SD), or progressive disease (PR). The median PFS rates were 29 weeks in PR, 16 weeks in SD, and 4 weeks in PR, respectively. Similarly, when a single [F-18] FDG PET positive/negative was considered after 4 weeks of sunitinib, the median PFS was 29 weeks for SUVs less than 8 g/mL versus 4 weeks for SUVs of 8 g/mL or greater. Multivariate analysis showed shorter PFS in patients who had higher residual SUVs and PFS was correlated with early [F-18] FDG PET metabolic response [28].

4.6 Conclusion

Despite computed tomography (CT) and magnetic resonance imaging (MRI) are well-accepted methods for diagnosis and staging of GISTs, the findings obtained from these modalities are not specific. However, several papers reported the CT and MRI features indicating a benign and malignant tendency.

Although GISTs also show non-specific findings on [F-18] FDG PET, it has a significant role in monitoring tumor response during imatinib and sunitinib therapy. The prognosis of GIST patients has a high correlation with the remnant and decrease of SUV values. Especially, it is useful to be able to evaluate tumor response to therapy at an early stage.

Acknowledgments This work was supported in part by grants from Scientific Research Expenses for Health and Welfare Programs, the Grant-in-Aid for Cancer Research from the Ministry of Health, Labor and Welfare, No. 15K09885, the Scientific Research Expenses for Health and Welfare Programs, No. 29-A-3 (Takashi Terauchi and Ukihide Tateishi: squad leaders), Practical Research for Innovative Cancer Control and Project Promoting Clinical Trials for Development of New Drugs by Japan Agency for Medical Research and Development (AMED).

References

1. Mazur MT, Clark HB. Gastric stromal tumors. Reappraisal of histogenesis. Am J Surg Pathol. 1983;7:507–19.
2. Kindblom LG, Remotti HE, Aldenborg F, et al. Gastrointestinal pacemaker cell tumor (GIPACT): gastrointestinal stromal tumors show phenotypic characteristics of the interstitial cells of Cajal. Am J Pathol. 1998;152:1259–69.
3. Hirota S, et al. Effects of loss-of-function and gain-of-function mutations of c-kit on the gastrointestinal tract. J Gastroenterol. 2000;35:75–9.
4. Subramanian S, West RB, Corless CL, et al. Gastrointestinal stromal tumors (GISTs) with KIT and PDGFRA mutations have distinct gene expression profiles. Oncogene. 2004;23:7780.
5. Sakurai S, Hasegawa T, Sakuma Y, et al. Myxoid epithelioid gastrointestinal stromal tumor (GIST) with mast cell infiltrations: a subtype of GIST with mutations of platelet-derived growth factor receptor alpha gene. Hum Pathol. 2004;35:1223–30.
6. Hirota S, Ohashi A, Nishida T, et al. Gain-of-function mutations of platelet-derived growth factor receptor alpha gene in gastrointestinal stromal tumors. Gastroenterology. 2003;125:660–7.
7. Sandrasegaran K, Rajesh A, Rushing DA, et al. Gastrointenstinal stromal tumors: CT and MRI findings. Eur Radiol. 2005;15:1407–14.
8. Ghanem N, Altehoefer C, Furtwangler A, et al. Computed tomography in gastrointestinal stromal tumors. Eur Radiol. 2003;13:1669–78.
9. Horton KM, Juluru K, Montogomery E, et al. Computed tomography imaging of gastrointestinal stromal tumors with pathology correlation. J Comput Assist Tomogr. 2004;28:811–7.
10. Kim HC, Lee JM, Kim SH, et al. Small gastrointestinal stromal tumours with focal areas of low attenuation on CT: pathological correlation. Clin Radiol. 2005;60:384–8.
11. Takao H, Yamahira K, Doi I, et al. Gastrointestinal stromal tumor of the retroperitoneum: CT and MR findings. Eur Radiol. 2004;14:1926–9.
12. Levy AD, Remotti HE, Thompson WM, Sobin LH, Miettinen M. Gastrointestinal stromal tumors: radiologic features with pathologic correlation. RadioGraphics. 2003;23:283–30.
13. Burkill GJ, Badran M, Al-Muderis O, et al. Malignant gastrointestinal stromal tumor: distribution, imaging features, and pattern of metastatic spread. Radiology. 2003;226:527–32.

14. Tateishi U, Hasegawa T, Satake M, et al. Gastrointestinal stromal tumor. Correlation of computed tomography findings with tumor grade and mortality. J Comput Assist Tomogr. 2003;27:792–8.
15. Yu MH, Lee JM, Baek JH, et al. MRI features of gastrointestinal stromal tumors. Am J Roentgenol. 2014;203(5):980–91.
16. Tateishi U, Miyake M, Maeda T, et al. CT and MRI findings in KIT-weak or KIT-negative atypical gastrointestinal stromal tumors. Eur Radiol. 2006;16:1537–43.
17. Miyake KK, Nakamoto Y, Mikami Y, et al. The predictive value of preoperative 18F-fluorodeoxyglucose PET for postoperative recurrence in patients with localized primary gastrointestinal stromal tumour. Eur Radiol. 2016;26:4664–74.
18. Patnaik S, Jyotsnarani Y, Rammurti S. Radiological features of metastatic gastrointestinal stromal tumor. J Clin Imaging Sci. 2012;2:43.
19. Katz SC, Dematteo RP. GISTS and leiomyosarcoma. J Surg Oncol. 2008;97:350–9.
20. Kong SH, Yang HK. Surgical treatment of gastric gastrointestinal tumor. J Gastric Cancer. 2013;13:3–18.
21. Tashiro T, Hasegawa T, Omatsu M, et al. Gastrointestinal stromal tumor of the stomach showing lymph node metastases. Histopathology. 2005;47:438–9.
22. van der Zwan SM, De Matteo RP. Gastrointestinal stromal tumor. 5 years later. Cancer. 2005;104:1781–8.
23. Agaimy A, Peter H. Lymph node metastasis in gastrointestinal stromal tumours (GIST) occurs preferentially in young patients ≤40 years: an overview based on our case material and the literature. Langenbeck's Arch Surg. 2009;394:375.
24. Gong N, Wong CS, Chu YC. Is lymph node metastasis a common feature of gastrointestinal stromal tumor? PET/CT correlation. Clin Nucl Med. 2011;36:678–82.
25. Gayed I, Vu T, Iyer R, et al. The role of 18F-FDG PET in staging and early prediction of response to therapy of recurrent gastrointestinal stromal tumors. J Nucl Med. 2004;45:17–21.
26. Choi H, Charnsangavej C, Faria SC, et al. Correlation of computed tomography and positron emission tomography in patients with metastatic gastrointestinal stromal tumor treated at a single institution with imatinib mesylate: proposal of new computed tomography response criteria. J Clin Oncol. 2007;25:1753–9.
27. Fuster D, Ayuso JR, Poveda A, et al. Value of FDG-PET for monitoring treatment response in patients with advanced GIST refractory to high-dose imatinib. A multicenter GEIS study. Q J Nucl Med Mol Imaging. 2011;55:680–7.
28. Prior JO, Montemurro M, Orcurto MV, et al. Early prediction of response to sunitinib after imatinib failure by 18F-fluorodeoxyglucose positron emission tomography in patients with gastrointestinal stromal tumor. J Clin Oncol. 2009;27:439–45.

5 Risk Classification

Hirotoshi Kikuchi, Hiroyuki Konno, and Hiroya Takeuchi

Abstract

Because postoperative recurrence or metastasis can occur even after complete resection of primary gastrointestinal stromal tumors (GISTs), adjuvant imatinib therapy with imatinib mesylate is recommended for patients who are at high risk of such recurrence. Classification of risk of GIST recurrence has recently become increasingly important in informing precise application of adjuvant therapy and prediction of overall outcome. Several risk-stratification systems, including the National Institutes of Health (NIH) consensus criteria, Armed Forces Institute of Pathology (AFIP) criteria, modified NIH criteria, contour maps, and prognostic nomograms, have been developed, based mainly on tumor size, mitotic counts, and primary site. Mutations in *c-kit* and *PDGFRA* genes and other genetic and epigenetic events appear to contribute to the malignant phenotype of GISTs. Of the currently available risk-stratification systems, the modified NIH criteria appear to be the best for selecting patients for whom postoperative adjuvant imatinib is indicated; however, even these criteria have some limitations and outstanding issues. Further studies aimed at improving available risk-stratification systems and thus enabling more precise identification of patients at high risk of recurrence for whom postoperative adjuvant imatinib is indicated are needed.

Keywords

NIH consensus criteria · Modified NIH criteria · AFIP criteria · Contour map · Nomogram

H. Kikuchi (✉) · H. Takeuchi
Department of Surgery, Hamamatsu University School of Medicine, Hamamatsu, Japan
e-mail: kikuchih@hama-med.ac.jp

H. Konno
Hamamatsu University School of Medicine, Hamamatsu, Japan

Y. Kurokawa, Y. Komatsu (eds.), *Gastrointestinal Stromal Tumor*,
https://doi.org/10.1007/978-981-13-3206-7_5

5.1 Introduction

Gastrointestinal stromal tumors (GISTs), which originate from the interstitial cells of Cajal (ICC) or their progenitor cells, are the commonest mesenchymal neoplasms of the human digestive tract [1, 2]. The current consensus is that gain-of-function mutations in the *c-kit* or platelet-derived growth factor receptor alpha (*PDGFRA*) genes in ICC are the leading cause of GISTs; such mutations result in ligand-independent activation of receptors, which in turn leads to tumor development and progression [3–5]. GISTs can arise in various parts of the gastrointestinal tract, most commonly in the stomach (60%), jejunum and ileum (30%), and duodenum and colorectum (5%) [6]. Their clinical aggressiveness can be evaluated on the basis of reported risk classification criteria [7–9]. Of these criteria, tumor size, mitotic count, and tumor site are regarded as the key factors most strongly impacting the prognosis of patients with GISTs.

Surgery is considered the most consistently effective treatment for primary GISTs; however, postoperative recurrence or metastasis reportedly occurs in 40–90% of patients whose primary GISTs have been treated by surgery alone [10, 11]. Recent clinical studies have demonstrated that adjuvant therapy with imatinib mesylate (Glivec®, Gleevec®; Novartis, Basel, Switzerland) can prolong recurrence-free survival (RFS) and overall survival (OS) in patients who are at high risk for GIST recurrence following resection [12–15]. However, the vast majority of patients with low-risk GISTs and therefore favorable outcomes after resection should not receive adjuvant imatinib therapy because of its high cost and risk of adverse events. In the current era of tyrosine kinase inhibitors (TKIs), classification of risk of GIST recurrence has become increasingly important in informing precise application of adjuvant therapy and prediction of overall outcome.

In this chapter, currently available risk classification strategies for prediction of GIST recurrence and provision of practical guidance in selecting patients for adjuvant imatinib therapy are described, and limitations and ongoing issues with these systems discussed.

5.2 Risk-Stratification Systems

5.2.1 National Institutes of Health (NIH) Consensus Criteria

The first risk-stratification system, which was developed by Fletcher et al. in 2002, is based mainly on the personal experience of an expert panel and known as the NIH consensus criteria (Table 5.1) [7]. These criteria classify risk of recurrence as very low, low, intermediate, or high on the basis of the two pathological variables of tumor size and mitotic count. According to these criteria, there are no benign GISTs; rather, the least malignant tumors are defined as very low risk. As this risk-stratification system incorporates only two variables, it is easily applicable and therefore a useful clinical tool; however, there are some issues regarding

Table 5.1 NIH consensus criteria

Risk category	Tumor size (cm)	Mitotic count (per 50 HPF)
Very low risk	<2	<5
Low risk	2–5	<5
Intermediate risk	<5	6–10
	5–10	<5
High risk	>5	>5
	>10	Any mitotic rate
	Any size	>10

Adapted with permission from Fletcher [7]
HPF high-power field

precise evaluation of risk of recurrence. Tumors with exactly five mitoses per 50 high-power fields (HPF) are not well-defined; additionally, this system does not take the anatomic site of the tumor or the presence of tumor rupture into consideration.

5.2.2 Armed Forces Institute of Pathology (AFIP) Criteria

The AFIP criteria were developed by Miettenen et al. using a large dataset from patients with GISTs in different parts of the gastrointestinal tract, 1765 in the stomach and 906 in the jejunum and ileum, and long-term follow-up [8, 16, 17]. These criteria incorporate the anatomic site of the primary tumor, tumor size, and mitotic count. Tumor size is categorized into four groups (≤2 cm, >2 to ≤5 cm, >5 to ≤10 cm, and >10 cm), mitotic count into two groups: ≤5 or >5 mitoses per 50 HPF, and tumor site as stomach, duodenum, ileum/jejunum, and rectum. These three variables are used to classify tumors into eight subgroups (Groups 1–6b) that correspond with five risk groups: none, very low, low, moderate, and high (Table 5.2). Even after surgical resection, patients with GISTs arising from the small bowel or rectum are at markedly higher risk of recurrence than those with gastric GISTs. Whereas the NIH consensus criteria classify all GISTs into four groups with at least some, albeit very low risk, the AFIP criteria include benign GISTs. For example, gastric GISTs less than 2 cm in diameter with fewer than five mitoses per 50 HPFs are categorized as benign GISTs with no risk of recurrence (Table 5.2). The AFIP criteria have the advantage of numerically estimating the risk of tumor relapse and/or progression during follow-up. However, this risk classification system does have some limitations in that it was developed from data of patients attending a single center. Additionally, this classification system does not recognize tumor rupture as a prognostic factor and incorporates only one cut-off value for mitotic count, which can result in substantially different risk estimations for GISTs with mitotic counts close to five per 50 HPFs. The complexity of these criteria with their eight prognostic subgroups may prejudice the sensitivity and specificity of prediction of recurrence.

Table 5.2 AFIP criteria

Group	Tumor size (cm)	Mitotic count (per 50 HPF)	Stomach	Small intestine	Duodenum	Rectum
1	≤2	≤5/50	None (0%)	None (0%)	None (0%)	None (0%)
2	>2 to ≤5		Very low (1.9%)	Low (4.3%)	Low (8.3%)	Low (8.5%)
3a	>5 to ≤10		Low (3.6%)	Moderate (24%)	Insufficient data	Insufficient data
3b	>10		Moderate (12%)	High (52%)	High (34%)	High (57%)
4	≤2	>5/50	None (0%)	High (50%)	Insufficient data	High (54%)
5	>2 to ≤5		Moderate (16%)	High (73%)	High (50%)	High (52%)
6a	>5 to ≤10		High (55%)	High (85%)	Insufficient data	Insufficient data
6b	>10		High (86%)	High (90%)	High (86%)	High (71%)

Adapted with permission from Miettinen and Lasota [8]
HPF high-power field

5.2.3 Modified NIH Criteria (Joensuu Risk Criteria)

The original NIH criteria developed by Fletcher et al. have some issues and limitations regarding patient selection for adjuvant therapy: they do not incorporate tumor site or tumor rupture, both of which have impacts on patient survival, and do not define risk classification of GISTs with exactly five mitoses per 50 HPFs. Joensuu therefore developed a modified version of the NIH risk classification system that adds the prognostic factors of primary tumor site and tumor rupture to the original NIH consensus criteria (Table 5.3) [9]. Tumor rupture is included as a high-risk factor for GISTs regardless of tumor size, mitotic count, or primary site. GISTs arising from organs other than stomach are categorized as moderate or high risk because non-gastric GISTs have a higher risk of recurrence. Another significant difference between this system and the NIH consensus criteria is classification of small (≤5 cm) non-gastric GISTs with more than five mitoses per 50 HPF and non-gastric GISTs of diameter between 5.1 and 10 cm and fewer than five mitoses per 50 HPFs, both of which are categorized as having high risk of recurrence in the modified NIH criteria [9]. Accordingly, some individuals who would be assigned to the intermediate risk group of the NIH consensus criteria are re-classified as being in the high risk group in the modified NIH criteria.

Joensuu et al. compared the three conventional risk-stratification systems described above by performing a pooled analysis of 2560 patients from 10 studies who had undergone surgery alone for GIST without adjuvant therapy [18]. The NIH consensus, modified NIH, and AFIP criteria were all strongly associated with RFS in the pooled dataset and the validation series (Fig. 5.1). In both datasets, the

Table 5.3 Modified NIH criteria

Risk category	Tumor size (cm)	Mitotic count (per 50 HPF)	Primary tumor site
Very low risk	<2.0	≤5	Any
Low risk	2.1–5.0	≤5	Any
Intermediate risk	2.1–5.0	>5	Gastric
	<5.0	6–10	Any
	5.1–10.0	≤5	Gastric
High risk	Any	Any	Tumor rupture
	>10	Any	Any
	Any	>10	Any
	>5.0	>5	Any
	2.1–5.0	>5	Non-gastric
	5.1–10.0	≤5	Non-gastric

Adapted with permission from Joensuu [9]
HPF high-power field

modified NIH criteria were the best for identifying a single high-risk group (Fig. 5.1c, d), whereas the AFIP criteria produced subgroups with RFS varying from very good to unfavorable (Fig. 5.1e, f). In a randomized trial of patients with macroscopically completely excised, KIT-positive GISTs and high risk of recurrence according to the modified NIH criteria, the Scandinavian Sarcoma Group (SSG) XVIII/Arbeitsgemeinschaft Internistische Onkologie (AIO) found that 3 years of adjuvant imatinib was significantly better than 1 year in extending RFS and OS [13, 14]. The modified consensus criteria are the most useful for selecting patients for whom postoperative adjuvant imatinib is indicated. Details of adjuvant therapy are described in Chap. 10. In contrast, the AFIP criteria are useful in that they incorporate molecular markers determined by immunohistochemical study of resected GISTs for predicting survival and provide a numerical estimate of the risk of recurrence and malignant potential (Table 5.2) [8].

5.2.4 Contour Maps

Joensuu et al. developed a new method for risk estimation using population-based cohorts of patients with operable GISTs who had not received adjuvant therapy [18]. Using continuous non-linear modeling of tumor size and mitotic count and incorporating tumor site and rupture, they generated novel prognostic contour maps (Fig. 5.2). The contour maps comprise nine maps according to tumor rupture status (with rupture, without rupture, and unknown), and tumor site (gastric, non-gastric, and extra-gastrointestinal). The percentages specified for each color indicate the probability of GIST recurrence within the first 10 years of follow-up after surgery. For example, the middle map of the left column (Fig. 5.2d) shows that the 10-year risk of GIST recurrence in a patient who had a 10 cm gastric GIST with five mitoses per 50 HPFs and no rupture is 20–40% [18].

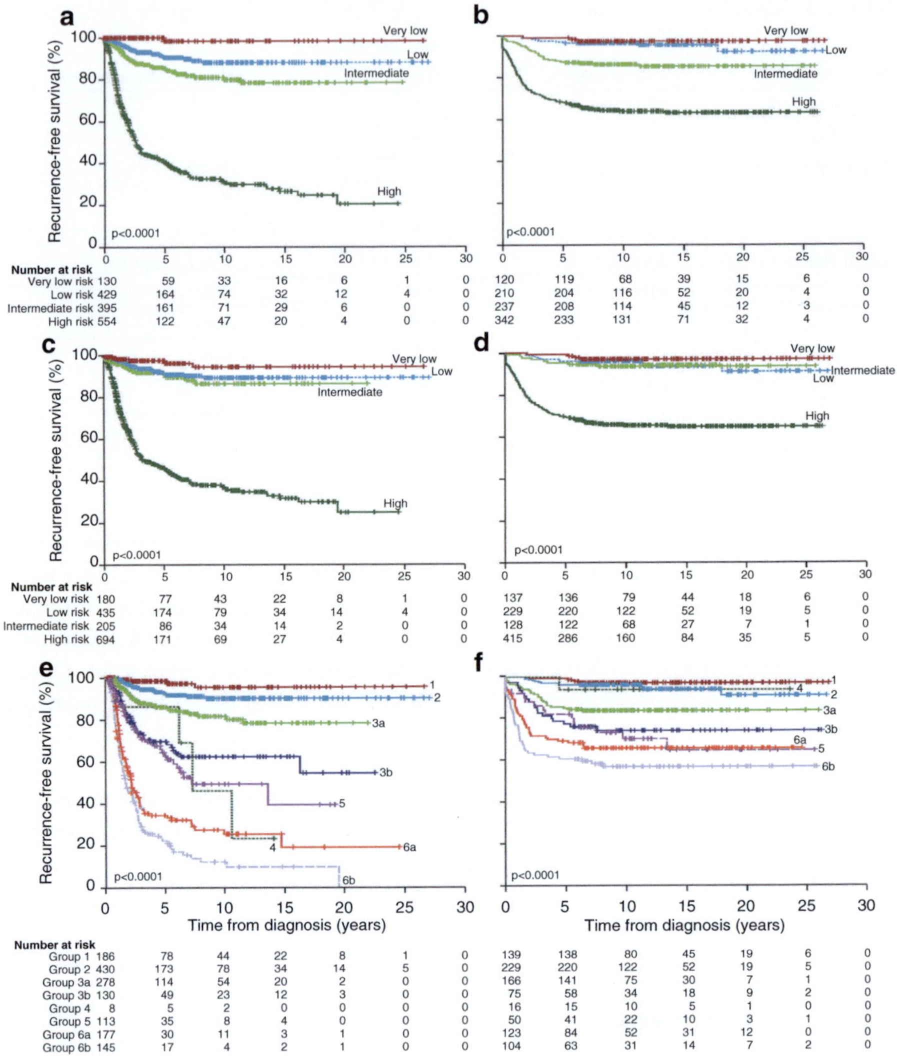

Fig. 5.1 Recurrence-free survival stratified by the National Institutes of Health (NIH) consensus criteria (**a**, **b**), modified NIH consensus criteria (**c**, **d**), and Armed Forces Institute of Pathology (AFIP) criteria (**e**, **f**). Panels **a**, **c**, **e** show pooled population-based series; panels **b**, **d**, **f** show validation series. Adapted with permission from Joensuu et al. [18]

In this report, Joensuu et al. used receiver operating characteristic (ROC) analyses to evaluate the prognostic accuracy of the non-linear models and conventional risk-stratification systems and found that the prognostic accuracy of the non-linear models was superior to those of the conventional risk-stratification schemes. In estimating the 10-year risk of GIST recurrence, the area under the curve (AUC) was larger for the non-linear model that included tumor rupture data (0.88, 95% CI 0.86–0.90) than for the NIH consensus criteria (0.79, 0.76–0.81; $p < 0.0001$),

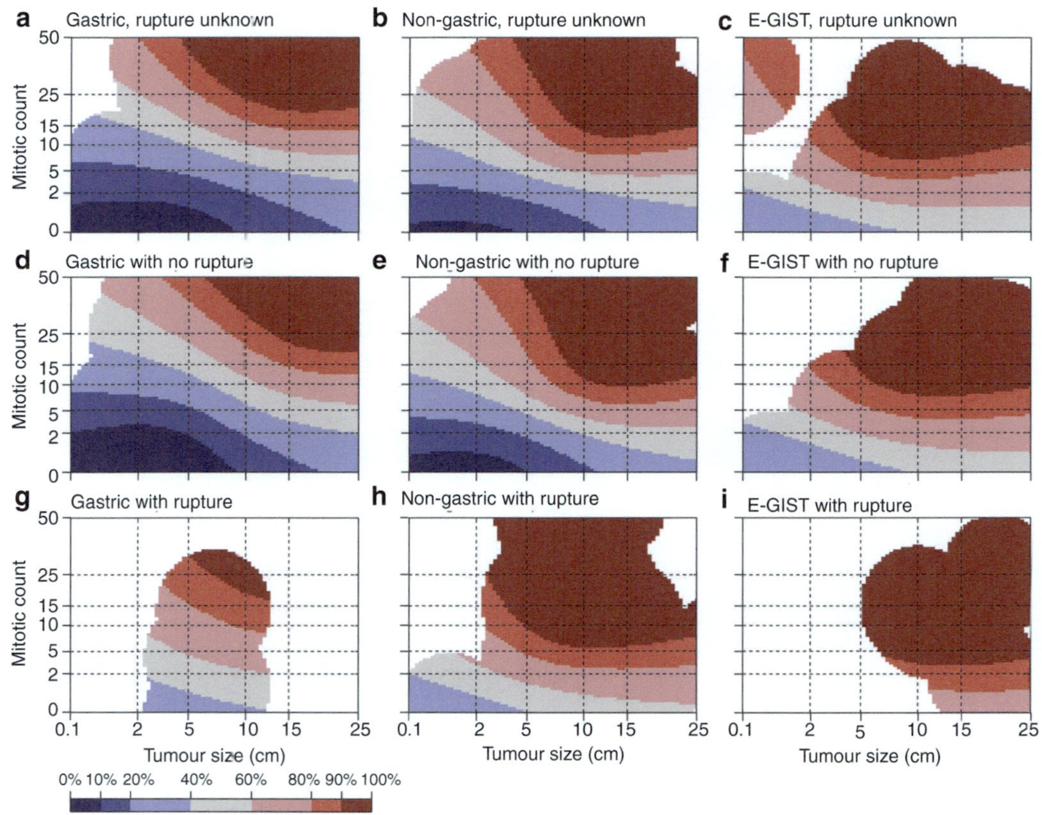

Fig. 5.2 Contour maps for estimating the risk of GIST recurrence after surgery. The maps in the top row are used when tumor rupture status is unknown (**a**–**c**), in the middle row when the tumor has not ruptured (**d**–**f**), and in the bottom row when tumor rupture has occurred (**g**–**i**). Red denotes high risk, blue low risk, and white lack of data. The percentages associated with each color (key) indicate the probability of GIST recurrence within the first 10 postoperative years. E-GIST, extra-gastrointestinal stromal tumor. Adapted with permission from Joensuu et al. [18]

modified NIH criteria (0.78, 0.75–0.80; $p < 0.0001$), AFIP criteria (0.82; 0.80–0.85; $p < 0.0001$), or non-linear model that did not include tumor rupture data (0.87, 0.85–0.89; $p = 0.005$) [18]. These data indicate that these contour maps are more accurate than the conventional risk-stratification systems in estimating the risk of GIST recurrence after surgery in patients who had only one GIST and did not have recurrent GIST or detectable metastases at the time of the diagnosis.

Although the contour maps are a reliable and useful means of risk classification for gastric, non-gastric, and extra-gastrointestinal GISTs with or without tumor rupture, several issues should be kept in mind when using this system in a clinical setting. The contour maps are not designed for selecting patients with GIST who are likely to benefit from adjuvant imatinib therapy and were not used in any randomized control trials that evaluated the benefits of adjuvant therapy. Although the contour maps enable estimation of the probability of GIST recurrence within the first 10 years after surgery, in Joensuu et al.'s pooled analysis most recurrences occurred within the first 5 years and few recurrences occurred from 10 years to 19.4 years after surgery [18]. The contour maps mainly show relatively short-term outcomes after surgery whereas late recurrence of GISTs is not rare.

5.2.5 Prognostic Nomograms

Gold et al. and Rossi et al. have each proposed a nomogram for estimating the risk of tumor progression after resection of GISTs [19, 20].

Gold et al.'s nomogram predicts 2- and 5-year RFS and was developed on the basis of tumor size (in cm), location (stomach, small intestine, colon/rectum, or other), and mitotic count (<5 or ≥5 mitoses per 50 HPFs) in a dataset of 127 patients who had been treated at Memorial Sloan-Kettering Cancer Center (Fig. 5.3) [19]. This nomogram was then validated in two external cohorts of patients from the Spanish national registry ($n = 212$) and Mayo Clinic ($n = 148$). The nomogram was evaluated both by calculating concordance probabilities and by testing calibration of predicted RFS with observed RFS. Concordance probabilities were also compared with those of three commonly employed staging systems. Concordance probabilities of the nomogram were superior to those of the NIH consensus and modified NIH criteria and equivalent to the AFIP criteria. Nomogram predictions of RFS appeared to be better calibrated than predictions made using the AFIP criteria [19].

Rossi et al. developed a nomogram by retrospective analysis of 929 GISTs resected at 35 Italian institutions between 1980 and 2000 [20]; 526 of these patients were found to be suitable for refining risk assessment by such a nomogram. This nomogram is also based on tumor size, mitotic count, and tumor site; however, tumor size and mitotic count are included as continuous variables, whereas the nomogram developed by Gold et al. categorizes mitotic count as either ≤5 or >5 mitoses per 50 HPFs [19, 20]. Although Rossi et al.'s nomogram can be used to predict OS, it has not been externally validated. Additionally, in contrast to Gold et al.'s nomogram, Rossi et al.'s nomogram cannot be used to predict RFS because these researchers lacked complete information on recurrence.

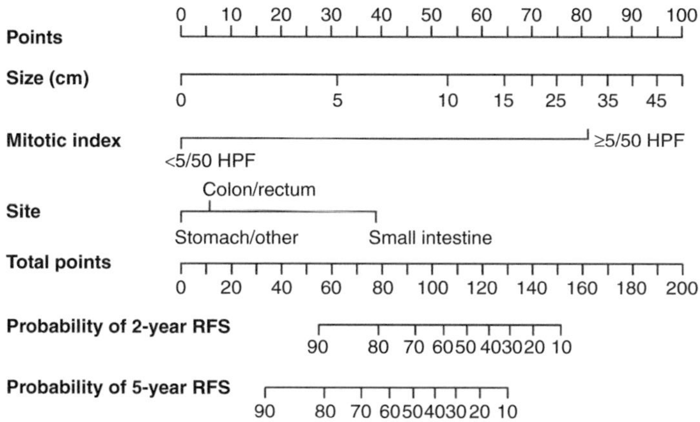

Fig. 5.3 Nomogram for predicting the probabilities of 2- and 5-year recurrence-free survival (RFS). Points are assigned for size, mitotic index, and site of origin by drawing a line upward from the corresponding values to the "Points" line. The sum of these three points plotted on the "Total Points" line corresponds to predictions of 2- and 5-year RFS. Adapted with permission from Gold et al. [19]

5.2.6 *C-kit* and *PDGFRA* Gene Mutations

Although gain-of-function mutations in the *c-kit* and *PDGFRA* genes are the main causes of GISTs, these genes also reportedly have prognostic or predictive implications. In 1998, Ernst et al. reported an association between *c-kit* mutation in gastrointestinal stromal/smooth muscle tumors and decreased survival [21]. In 1999, Taniguchi et al. reported that mutation-positive GISTs have more mitotic figures and more necrosis and hemorrhage than GISTs without mutations and that *c-kit* mutation is an independent prognostic factor for OS and cause-specific survival [22]. In 2004, Kim et al. reported that tumors with c-*kit* mutations have higher mitotic counts and cellularity than those without these mutations and that multivariate analyses revealed an association between poor RFS and the presence of *c-kit* mutations [23]. In 2002, Singer et al. reported that the presence of c-*kit* exon 11 deletion or insertion is an adverse independent prognostic factor for disease-free survival (DFS) [24]. In 2005 and 2006, a significant correlation between deletions affecting codons 557–558 of *c-kit* and poor RFS was reported [25–27]. GISTs with *c-kit* exon 9 duplication reportedly behave more aggressively than those without such duplication [28]. There is also reportedly an association between GISTs with a D842V substitution in exon 18, the most common *PDGFRA* gene mutation, and gastric GISTs, epithelioid morphology, and a less malignant course of disease [8, 28]. These reports indicate the prognostic importance of *c-kit* and *PDGFRA* mutations in GISTs. However, most of these data on the impacts of *c-kit* and *PDGFRA* mutations on patients' prognosis were reported before TKIs were widely used for recurrent GISTs or in the adjuvant setting, which significantly affects patients' survival.

In the era of TKIs, it is also important to consider the differential effects of *c-kit* and *PDGFRA* mutations on responses to TKIs administered for recurrent GISTs and in the adjuvant setting. For example, GISTs harboring primary mutations at codons 557–558 of the *c-kit* gene, which have been reported to indicate a poor prognosis, are likely to respond well to imatinib [25–27]. GISTs harboring *PDGFRA* mutation D842V reportedly have a relatively favor prognosis; however, these tumors are resistant to imatinib [8, 28–30]. Further analysis in other large series with long-term follow-up is required to better evaluate the roles of mutational status in GIST risk-stratification systems.

5.2.7 Other Pathological Variables and Molecular Markers

There are some reports on the prognostic implication of pathologic variables other than tumor size and mitotic count in GISTs. Hasegawa et al. investigated the clinicopathological features of 171 GISTs that were surgically resected in a single institution and proposed a histologic grading system using tumor differentiation, Ki-67 (MIB-1) score, and necrosis [31]. In their study, multivariate analysis showed that both tumor size >10 cm and high grade were significantly associated with a poor outcome. On the basis of their data, they classified GISTs >10 cm or high grade, 5–10 cm and low grade, and ≤5 cm and low grade are high risk, intermediate risk, and low risk for mortality, respectively [31]. Liu et al. performed a large-scale multicenter retrospective analysis to determine the clinical utility of tumor necrosis in patients undergoing curative resection for gastric GIST. In their study, multivariate analysis revealed that tumor necrosis was an independent predictor of unfavorable DFS [32].

Tumor angiogenesis plays important roles in growth and metastasis and vascular endothelial growth factor (VEGF) plays a central role in promoting tumor angiogenesis in various kinds of solid tumors, including gastrointestinal cancers such as gastric and colon cancers [33–36]. Hypoxia inducible factor (HIF)-1α, which activates expression of VEGFA, is a master regulator of hypoxia responses [37, 38]. Takahashi et al. immunohistochemically analyzed VEGF and Ki-67 expression, microvessel density (MVD), and HIF-1α in 53 GISTs and identified by multiple logistic regression analysis that VEGF expression and high mitotic rate are independent predictors of poor 10-year survival. They found that prognosis was significantly poorer in patients with GISTs expressing HIF-1α than in those whose GISTs lacked HIF-1α expression [39, 40]. Imamura et al. investigated the role of angiogenesis in 95 GISTs by immunohistochemical analysis for MVD and VEGF expression and identified by multivariate analysis that tumor grade and MVD are independent prognostic factors [41]. The important roles of angiogenesis in the progression of GIST were subsequently confirmed by other studies elsewhere [42, 43]. Although tumor angiogenesis appears to play an important role in progression of GIST, further studies are needed to evaluate whether pathological variables such as MVD and VEGF expression can be used to predict the postoperative prognosis of patients with GIST.

Approximately, 10–15% of GISTs do not carry mutations in *c-kit* or *PDGFRA*, and are referred to as wild-type (WT) GISTs. About half of WT GISTs show loss of function of the succinate dehydrogenase complex (SDH), and those tumors are designated as SDH-deficient or SDHB-negative GISTs based on their immunohistochemical status [44, 45]. SDH enzyme dysfunction leads to accumulation of succinate, resulting in HIF1-α stabilization. SDH-deficient GISTs have distinctive clinicopathological features; are found mainly in children and in younger adults, show an epithelioid or mixed histologic subtype, and show an indolent course of disease whereas frequently metastasize to lymph nodes [46, 47].

Many researchers have used a variety of approaches, including genomics, proteomics, and bioinformatics, in their attempts to identify novel molecular markers for predicting prognosis of patients with GISTs. A microsatellite analysis showed that deletion of Hox11L1 is associated with a poor prognosis [48]. Yamaguchi et al. performed microarray analyses in 32 primary GISTs and immunohistochemical analysis of 152 gastric GISTs and reported that dipeptidyl peptidase IV (T-cell activation antigen CD26) protein is significantly associated with poor OS and DFS [49]. Suehara et al. used two-dimensional difference gel electrophoresis to analyze protein expression profiles. Comparing these profiles between GISTs with good and poor prognoses resulted in identification of potassium channel tetramerization domain-containing 12 (KCTD12), also known as pfetin, as a protein that discriminates between these two groups and which they found to be a useful and reliable biomarker for both the diagnosis and prognosis of GIST [50, 51]. Setoguchi et al. performed microarray analysis to compare gene expression profiles between primary gastric and metastatic liver GISTs and identified high expression of versican and loss of CD9 as potential prognostic markers for gastric GISTs [52]. Using multivariate analysis, Yen et al. identified aurora kinase A (AURKA), which encodes a mitotic centrosomal protein kinase, as an independent unfavorable prognostic factor for RFS [53, 54]. Yamamoto et al. analyzed microRNA (miRNA) expression profiles by miRNA array in 19 GISTs and identified miR-133b as being downregulated in high-grade GISTs. They found that high concentrations of the protein fascin-1, a negative target of miR-133b, correlated significantly with shorter DFS [55]. Bertucci et al. searched for a gene expression signature (GES) that predicts RFS and compared its performance to those of three published prognostic proliferation-based GES (Genomic Grade Index [GGI], 16-kinase, and CINSARC) and the AFIP classification [56]. They found that the GGI splits the AFIP intermediate/high-risk categories into two groups with different outcomes, suggesting that GES may be a promising new method for estimating the risk of GIST recurrence [56]. Recent studies demonstrated the clinical utility of liquid biopsies in cancer diagnosis and precision medicine. Molecular analysis of circulating tumor DNA (ctDNA) has been investigated to detect mutations of *c-kit* and *PDGFRA* genes in GISTs. Although future studies with a large number of patients are needed, detection of ctDNA appears to have potential to become a major method to capture the molecular heterogeneity of the whole tumor that associates with tumor burden [57].

Thus far, no pathological variables other than mitotic count and molecular markers have been incorporated into GIST risk-stratification systems or widely used clinically. Although further studies with more data are needed, we expect molecular markers or mutational status of *c-kit* and *PDGFRA* genes to be incorporated into currently available risk-stratification systems to enable more precise identification of patients at high risk of recurrence for whom adjuvant imatinib is indicated.

5.3 Discussion

This chapter began with the introduction of three major risk-stratification systems, the NIH consensus, AFIP, and modified NIH criteria. Although those criteria are relatively simple and reliable and the most used clinically, they all have limitations, a major one being the cut-off points for mitotic count and tumor size. In particular, tumors with close to five mitoses per 50 HPFs can be evaluated as having markedly different risks of recurrence. Because cellularity and mitoses in GISTs are often heterogeneous and there is no consensus on cut-off for mitotic count, the evaluation of mitotic count can be subjective. Determination of tumor size is also sometimes problematic.

In the current era of TKIs, the most important purpose of the application of these criteria is to select patients for whom adjuvant imatinib therapy is indicated. Three years of adjuvant imatinib therapy is currently recommended for patients with GIST with high-risk features according to the modified NIH criteria, this recommendation being based on the reported survival benefits of adjuvant imatinib in randomized controlled trials [12–14, 58]. Trials to evaluate adjuvant imatinib therapy for longer than 3 years have now been initiated. Some outstanding issues remain regarding the optimal duration of adjuvant imatinib for high-risk patients after complete resection of GISTs. Although 3 years of adjuvant imatinib therapy resulted in longer survival than 1 year of imatinib in the SSG XVIII/AIO trial, about half of the patients had no recurrences even after stopping adjuvant imatinib. The 5-year survival rates of patients assigned to the 1-year group were also high (85.3% in intention-to-treat cohort) because their recurrences were treated with TKIs [14]. In this trial, although most patients tolerated imatinib relatively well, almost all had adverse events [14]. Additionally, the cost of adjuvant treatment with imatinib can also be problematic for patients with GISTs. Thus, the current patient selection criteria may result in overtreatment of patients with GISTs undergoing R0 resection. Development of a novel classification of risk of recurrence based on biological markers is expected to further improve selection criteria for patients to receive adjuvant therapy.

In the currently available risk-stratification systems, the modified NIH criteria seem to be the best for selecting patients for whom adjuvant imatinib is indicated. However, the criteria do not reflect mutation status of the *c-kit* or *PDGFRA* genes. Indeed, none of the available risk-stratification systems incorporate mutation data. Considering the favorable outcome of GIST harboring codon D842V mutation at *PDFRA* gene and unfavorable outcome of tumors with *c-kit* exon 9 mutation or codons 557–558 at exon 11 of the *c-kit* gene [25–28], future studies should try to integrate tumor mutation status into prognostic criteria schemes. In addition, adjuvant imatinib therapy may modify the impacts of prognostic factors currently used in risk models.

Intestinal GISTs have markedly higher risks for post-resection recurrence than gastric GISTs [8, 9, 17, 18, 59]. Approximately 40–50% of intestinal GISTs are clinically malignant, whereas 20–25% of gastric GIST reportedly behave in an aggressive manner [59]. Generally, intestinal GISTs are difficult to diagnose before symptoms, such as gastrointestinal bleeding or an acute abdomen, develop and they tend to be larger by the time a diagnosis is made [59]. Although tumor size and mitotic count are considered the best predictors of prognosis in patients with GISTs, patients with intestinal GISTs still have a worse prognosis than those with gastric GISTs after matching them for size and mitotic count [8, 17, 18]. Thus far, the mechanisms underlying the malignant behavior of intestinal GISTs have not been well characterized. Hara et al. used microarrays to compare gene expression profiles of gastric, intestinal, and metastatic liver GISTs and found that the gene profiles of intestinal GISTs are similar to those of malignant and metastatic liver GISTs, but distinct from those of gastric GISTs [60]. These findings suggest that intestinal GISTs may express genes involved in the malignant transformation of GIST from early in their development.

Although activating mutations of the *c-kit* gene are the main cause of GISTs, several groups have reported a high incidence of small GISTs, known as occult or incidental GISTs, that carry a mutation in the *c-kit* gene [61, 62]. It seems that although *c-kit* gene mutation is the major event in the initiation of GIST, it alone is not sufficient; rather, substantial genetic changes other than in the *c-kit* gene or epigenetic changes being necessary for the development of clinical GISTs. Chromosomal alterations such as the loss of chromosome 14q and 22q have been reported in primary GISTs [63–66]. Occurrence of these chromosomal alterations in the early stages of GISTs may work as a second hit event leading to the development of a clinical GIST that may still be low risk. A third event seems to be involved in the development of malignant or metastatic GISTs. In Sect. 5.2.7, potential genetic or epigenetic changes other than *c-kit* gene and *PDGFRA* gene mutations that may regulate the biological behavior of GISTs are described. Incorporation of these molecular alterations may contribute to the evaluation of the prognoses of patients with GISTs. Future clinical, basic, and translational research is expected to improve the currently available risk-stratification criteria by incorporating molecular events involved in the malignant transformation of GISTs.

In conclusion, several risk classification criteria for GISTs based mainly on tumor size, mitotic counts, and primary site have been developed. Among the currently available risk-stratification systems, the modified NIH criteria appear to be the best for selecting patients for whom adjuvant imatinib is indicated; however, there are some limitations and outstanding issues. Future studies are expected to improve currently available risk-stratification systems, thus enabling more precise identification of patients at high risk.

Acknowledgment We thank Dr. Trish Reynolds, MBBS, FRACP, from Edanz Group (www.edanzediting.com/ac), for editing the English text of a draft of this chapter.

References

1. Kindblom LG, Remotti HE, Aldenborg F, Meis-Kindblom JM. Gastrointestinal pacemaker cell tumor (GIPACT): gastrointestinal stromal tumors show phenotypic characteristics of the interstitial cells of Cajal. Am J Pathol. 1998;152(5):1259–69.
2. O'Leary T, Berman JJ. Gastrointestinal stromal tumors: answers and questions. Hum Pathol. 2002;33(5):456–8.
3. Hirota S, Isozaki K, Moriyama Y, Hashimoto K, Nishida T, Ishiguro S, et al. Gain-of-function mutations of c-kit in human gastrointestinal stromal tumors. Science. 1998;279(5350):577–80.
4. Hirota S, Ohashi A, Nishida T, Isozaki K, Kinoshita K, Shinomura Y, et al. Gain-of-function mutations of platelet-derived growth factor receptor alpha gene in gastrointestinal stromal tumors. Gastroenterology. 2003;125(3):660–7.
5. Heinrich MC, Corless CL, Duensing A, McGreevey L, Chen CJ, Joseph N, et al. PDGFRA activating mutations in gastrointestinal stromal tumors. Science. 2003;299(5607):708–10.
6. Patil DT, Rubin BP. Gastrointestinal stromal tumor: advances in diagnosis and management. Arch Pathol Lab Med. 2011;135(10):1298–310.
7. Fletcher CD. Clinicopathologic correlations in gastrointestinal stromal tumors. Hum Pathol. 2002;33(5):455.
8. Miettinen M, Lasota J. Gastrointestinal stromal tumors: pathology and prognosis at different sites. Semin Diagn Pathol. 2006;23(2):70–83.
9. Joensuu H. Risk stratification of patients diagnosed with gastrointestinal stromal tumor. Hum Pathol. 2008;39(10):1411–9.
10. DeMatteo RP, Lewis JJ, Leung D, Mudan SS, Woodruff JM, Brennan MF. Two hundred gastrointestinal stromal tumors: recurrence patterns and prognostic factors for survival. Ann Surg. 2000;231(1):51–8.
11. Roberts PJ, Eisenberg B. Clinical presentation of gastrointestinal stromal tumors and treatment of operable disease. Eur J Cancer. 2002;38(Suppl 5):S37–8.
12. Dematteo RP, Ballman KV, Antonescu CR, Maki RG, Pisters PW, Demetri GD, et al. Adjuvant imatinib mesylate after resection of localised, primary gastrointestinal stromal tumour: a randomised, double-blind, placebo-controlled trial. Lancet. 2009;373(9669):1097–104.
13. Joensuu H, Eriksson M, Sundby Hall K, Hartmann JT, Pink D, Schutte J, et al. One vs three years of adjuvant imatinib for operable gastrointestinal stromal tumor: a randomized trial. JAMA. 2012;307(12):1265–72.
14. Joensuu H, Eriksson M, Sundby Hall K, Reichardt A, Hartmann JT, Pink D, et al. adjuvant imatinib for high-risk GI stromal tumor: analysis of a randomized trial. J Clin Oncol. 2016;34(3):244–50.
15. Casali PG, Le Cesne A, Poveda Velasco A, Kotasek D, Rutkowski P, Hohenberger P, et al. Time to definitive failure to the first tyrosine kinase inhibitor in localized GI stromal tumors treated with imatinib as an adjuvant: a European Organisation for Research and Treatment of Cancer Soft Tissue and Bone Sarcoma Group intergroup randomized trial in collaboration with the Australasian Gastro-Intestinal Trials Group, UNICANCER, French Sarcoma Group, Italian Sarcoma Group, and Spanish Group for Research on Sarcomas. J Clin Oncol. 2015;33(36):4276–83.
16. Miettinen M, Sobin LH, Lasota J. Gastrointestinal stromal tumors of the stomach: a clinicopathologic, immunohistochemical, and molecular genetic study of 1765 cases with long-term follow-up. Am J Surg Pathol. 2005;29(1):52–68.
17. Miettinen M, Makhlouf H, Sobin LH, Lasota J. Gastrointestinal stromal tumors of the jejunum and ileum: a clinicopathologic, immunohistochemical, and molecular genetic study of 906 cases before imatinib with long-term follow-up. Am J Surg Pathol. 2006;30(4):477–89.
18. Joensuu H, Vehtari A, Riihimaki J, Nishida T, Steigen SE, Brabec P, et al. Risk of recurrence of gastrointestinal stromal tumour after surgery: an analysis of pooled population-based cohorts. Lancet Oncol. 2012;13(3):265–74.
19. Gold JS, Gonen M, Gutierrez A, Broto JM, Garcia-del-Muro X, Smyrk TC, et al. Development and validation of a prognostic nomogram for recurrence-free survival after complete surgical

resection of localised primary gastrointestinal stromal tumour: a retrospective analysis. Lancet Oncol. 2009;10(11):1045–52.
20. Rossi S, Miceli R, Messerini L, Bearzi I, Mazzoleni G, Capella C, et al. Natural history of imatinib-naive GISTs: a retrospective analysis of 929 cases with long-term follow-up and development of a survival nomogram based on mitotic index and size as continuous variables. Am J Surg Pathol. 2011;35(11):1646–56.
21. Ernst SI, Hubbs AE, Przygodzki RM, Emory TS, Sobin LH, O'Leary TJ. KIT mutation portends poor prognosis in gastrointestinal stromal/smooth muscle tumors. Lab Invest. 1998;78(12):1633–6.
22. Taniguchi M, Nishida T, Hirota S, Isozaki K, Ito T, Nomura T, et al. Effect of c-kit mutation on prognosis of gastrointestinal stromal tumors. Cancer Res. 1999;59(17):4297–300.
23. Kim TW, Lee H, Kang YK, Choe MS, Ryu MH, Chang HM, et al. Prognostic significance of c-kit mutation in localized gastrointestinal stromal tumors. Clin Cancer Res. 2004;10(9):3076–81.
24. Singer S, Rubin BP, Lux ML, Chen CJ, Demetri GD, Fletcher CD, et al. Prognostic value of KIT mutation type, mitotic activity, and histologic subtype in gastrointestinal stromal tumors. J Clin Oncol. 2002;20(18):3898–905.
25. Martin J, Poveda A, Llombart-Bosch A, Ramos R, Lopez-Guerrero JA, Garcia del Muro J, et al. Deletions affecting codons 557-558 of the c-KIT gene indicate a poor prognosis in patients with completely resected gastrointestinal stromal tumors: a study by the Spanish Group for Sarcoma Research (GEIS). J Clin Oncol. 2005;23(25):6190–8.
26. Iesalnieks I, Rummele P, Dietmaier W, Jantsch T, Zulke C, Schlitt HJ, et al. Factors associated with disease progression in patients with gastrointestinal stromal tumors in the pre-imatinib era. Am J Clin Pathol. 2005;124(5):740–8.
27. Andersson J, Bumming P, Meis-Kindblom JM, Sihto H, Nupponen N, Joensuu H, et al. Gastrointestinal stromal tumors with KIT exon 11 deletions are associated with poor prognosis. Gastroenterology. 2006;130(6):1573–81.
28. Lasota J, Miettinen M. KIT and PDGFRA mutations in gastrointestinal stromal tumors (GISTs). Semin Diagn Pathol. 2006;23(2):91–102.
29. Debiec-Rychter M, Cools J, Dumez H, Sciot R, Stul M, Mentens N, et al. Mechanisms of resistance to imatinib mesylate in gastrointestinal stromal tumors and activity of the PKC412 inhibitor against imatinib-resistant mutants. Gastroenterology. 2005;128(2):270–9.
30. Heinrich MC, Corless CL, Demetri GD, Blanke CD, von Mehren M, Joensuu H, et al. Kinase mutations and imatinib response in patients with metastatic gastrointestinal stromal tumor. J Clin Oncol. 2003;21(23):4342–9.
31. Hasegawa T, Matsuno Y, Shimoda T, Hirohashi S. Gastrointestinal stromal tumor: consistent CD117 immunostaining for diagnosis, and prognostic classification based on tumor size and MIB-1 grade. Hum Pathol. 2002;33(6):669–76.
32. Liu X, Qiu H, Zhang P, Feng X, Chen T, Li Y, et al. Prognostic role of tumor necrosis in patients undergoing curative resection for gastric gastrointestinal stromal tumor: a multicenter analysis of 740 cases in China. Cancer Med. 2017;6(12):2796–803.
33. Folkman J. Angiogenesis in psoriasis: therapeutic implications. J Invest Dermatol. 1972;59(1):40–3.
34. Bergers G, Benjamin LE. Tumorigenesis and the angiogenic switch. Nat Rev Cancer. 2003;3(6):401–10.
35. Ferrara N, Davis-Smyth T. The biology of vascular endothelial growth factor. Endocr Rev. 1997;18(1):4–25.
36. Ferrara N. VEGF and the quest for tumour angiogenesis factors. Nat Rev Cancer. 2002;2(10):795–803.
37. Harris AL. Hypoxia – a key regulatory factor in tumour growth. Nat Rev Cancer. 2002;2(1):38–47.
38. Cummins EP, Taylor CT. Hypoxia-responsive transcription factors. Pflugers Arch Eur J Physiol. 2005;450(6):363–71.
39. Takahashi R, Tanaka S, Kitadai Y, Sumii M, Yoshihara M, Haruma K, et al. Expression of vascular endothelial growth factor and angiogenesis in gastrointestinal stromal tumor of the stomach. Oncology. 2003;64(3):266–74.

40. Takahashi R, Tanaka S, Hiyama T, Ito M, Kitadai Y, Sumii M, et al. Hypoxia-inducible factor-1alpha expression and angiogenesis in gastrointestinal stromal tumor of the stomach. Oncol Rep. 2003;10(4):797–802.
41. Imamura M, Yamamoto H, Nakamura N, Oda Y, Yao T, Kakeji Y, et al. Prognostic significance of angiogenesis in gastrointestinal stromal tumor. Mod Pathol. 2007;20(5):529–37.
42. Zhao Y, Wang Q, Deng X. Altered angiogenesis gene expression in gastrointestinal stromal tumors: potential use in diagnosis, outcome prediction, and treatment. Neoplasma. 2012;59(4):384–92.
43. Basilio-de-Oliveira RP, Pannain VL. Prognostic angiogenic markers (endoglin, VEGF, CD31) and tumor cell proliferation (Ki67) for gastrointestinal stromal tumors. World J Gastroenterol: WJG. 2015;21(22):6924–30.
44. Gill AJ, Chou A, Vilain R, Clarkson A, Lui M, Jin R, et al. Immunohistochemistry for SDHB divides gastrointestinal stromal tumors (GISTs) into 2 distinct types. Am J Surg Pathol. 2010;34(5):636–44.
45. Miettinen M, Wang ZF, Sarlomo-Rikala M, Osuch C, Rutkowski P, Lasota J. Succinate dehydrogenase-deficient GISTs: a clinicopathologic, immunohistochemical, and molecular genetic study of 66 gastric GISTs with predilection to young age. Am J Surg Pathol. 2011;35(11):1712–21.
46. Pantaleo MA, Lolli C, Nannini M, Astolfi A, Indio V, Saponara M, et al. Good survival outcome of metastatic SDH-deficient gastrointestinal stromal tumors harboring SDHA mutations. Genet Med. 2015;17(5):391–5.
47. Miettinen M, Killian JK, Wang ZF, Lasota J, Lau C, Jones L, et al. Immunohistochemical loss of succinate dehydrogenase subunit A (SDHA) in gastrointestinal stromal tumors (GISTs) signals SDHA germline mutation. Am J Surg Pathol. 2013;37(2):234–40.
48. Kaifi JT, Wagner M, Schurr PG, Wachowiak R, Reichelt U, Yekebas EF, et al. Allelic loss of Hox11L1 gene locus predicts outcome of gastrointestinal stromal tumors. Oncol Rep. 2006;16(4):915–9.
49. Yamaguchi U, Nakayama R, Honda K, Ichikawa H, Hasegawa T, Shitashige M, et al. Distinct gene expression-defined classes of gastrointestinal stromal tumor. J Clin Oncol. 2008;26(25):4100–8.
50. Suehara Y, Kondo T, Seki K, Shibata T, Fujii K, Gotoh M, et al. Pfetin as a prognostic biomarker of gastrointestinal stromal tumors revealed by proteomics. Clin Cancer Res. 2008;14(6):1707–17.
51. Hasegawa T, Asanuma H, Ogino J, Hirohashi Y, Shinomura Y, Iwaki H, et al. Use of potassium channel tetramerization domain-containing 12 as a biomarker for diagnosis and prognosis of gastrointestinal stromal tumor. Hum Pathol. 2013;44:1271–7.
52. Setoguchi T, Kikuchi H, Yamamoto M, Baba M, Ohta M, Kamiya K, et al. Microarray analysis identifies versican and CD9 as potent prognostic markers in gastric gastrointestinal stromal tumors. Cancer Sci. 2011;102(4):883–9.
53. Yen CC, Yeh CN, Cheng CT, Jung SM, Huang SC, Chang TW, et al. Integrating bioinformatics and clinicopathological research of gastrointestinal stromal tumors: identification of aurora kinase A as a poor risk marker. Ann Surg Oncol. 2012;19(11):3491–9.
54. Yeh CN, Yen CC, Chen YY, Cheng CT, Huang SC, Chang TW, et al. Identification of aurora kinase A as an unfavorable prognostic factor and potential treatment target for metastatic gastrointestinal stromal tumors. Oncotarget. 2014;5(12):4071–86.
55. Yamamoto H, Kohashi K, Fujita A, Oda Y. Fascin-1 overexpression and miR-133b downregulation in the progression of gastrointestinal stromal tumor. Mod Pathol. 2013;26(4):563–71.
56. Bertucci F, Finetti P, Ostrowski J, Kim WK, Kim H, Pantaleo MA, et al. Genomic Grade Index predicts postoperative clinical outcome of GIST. Br J Cancer. 2012;107(8):1433–41.
57. Namlos HM, Boye K, Mishkin SJ, Baroy T, Lorenz S, Bjerkehagen B, et al. Non-invasive detection of ctDNA reveals intratumour heterogeneity and is associated with tumour burden in gastrointestinal stromal tumour. Mol Cancer Ther. 2018;17:2473–80.

58. Joensuu H, Martin-Broto J, Nishida T, Reichardt P, Schoffski P, Maki RG. Follow-up strategies for patients with gastrointestinal stromal tumour treated with or without adjuvant imatinib after surgery. Eur J Cancer. 2015;51(12):1611–7.
59. Miettinen M, Lasota J. Gastrointestinal stromal tumors: review on morphology, molecular pathology, prognosis, and differential diagnosis. Arch Pathol Lab Med. 2006;130(10):1466–78.
60. Hara R, Kikuchi H, Setoguchi T, Miyazaki S, Yamamoto M, Hiramatsu Y, et al. Microarray analysis reveals distinct gene set profiles for gastric and intestinal gastrointestinal stromal tumors. Anticancer Res. 2015;35(6):3289–98.
61. Kawanowa K, Sakuma Y, Sakurai S, Hishima T, Iwasaki Y, Saito K, et al. High incidence of microscopic gastrointestinal stromal tumors in the stomach. Hum Pathol. 2006;37(12):1527–35.
62. Agaimy A, Wunsch PH, Hofstaedter F, Blaszyk H, Rummele P, Gaumann A, et al. Minute gastric sclerosing stromal tumors (GIST tumorlets) are common in adults and frequently show c-KIT mutations. Am J Surg Pathol. 2007;31(1):113–20.
63. Fukasawa T, Chong JM, Sakurai S, Koshiishi N, Ikeno R, Tanaka A, et al. Allelic loss of 14q and 22q, NF2 mutation, and genetic instability occur independently of c-kit mutation in gastrointestinal stromal tumor. Jpn J Cancer Res. 2000;91(12):1241–9.
64. Wozniak A, Sciot R, Guillou L, Pauwels P, Wasag B, Stul M, et al. Array CGH analysis in primary gastrointestinal stromal tumors: cytogenetic profile correlates with anatomic site and tumor aggressiveness, irrespective of mutational status. Genes Chromosom Cancer. 2007;46(3):261–76.
65. Chen Y, Tzeng CC, Liou CP, Chang MY, Li CF, Lin CN. Biological significance of chromosomal imbalance aberrations in gastrointestinal stromal tumors. J Biomed Sci. 2004;11(1):65–71.
66. Assamaki R, Sarlomo-Rikala M, Lopez-Guerrero JA, Lasota J, Andersson LC, Llombart-Bosch A, et al. Array comparative genomic hybridization analysis of chromosomal imbalances and their target genes in gastrointestinal stromal tumors. Genes Chromosom Cancer. 2007;46(6):564–76.

Treatment Guidelines

6

Muranaka Tetsuhito and Yoshito Komatsu

Abstract

A gastrointestinal stromal tumor (GIST) is one of the soft tissue neoplasms with malignant potential, and it requires complete resection for cure. Very small GISTs (<2 cm) without high-risk features on endoscopic ultrasonography can be placed under observation. For other resectable GISTs, complete resection should be initially considered. Postoperative imatinib administration for at least 36 months should be considered in patients with a significant risk of recurrence. Imatinib is recommended as the first-line treatment in patients with unresectable or metastatic GISTs. Sunitinib administration is recommended for imatinib-resistant GISTs. Regorafenib should be considered in patients with imatinib or sunitinib-resistant GISTs. During these tyrosine kinase therapies, surgery should be considered if feasible.

Keywords

Guideline · Principle · Treatment

6.1 Introduction

A gastrointestinal stromal tumor (GIST) is one of the soft tissue neoplasms with malignant potential, and it requires complete resection for cure. Most GISTs have a malignant potential, except benign and very small tumors, but the treatment strategy should be slightly different from that for cancer. According to the NCCN guidelines version 2.2018 [1], GISTs can be categorized as follows: very small gastric GISTs (<2 cm), localized or potentially resectable GISTs, and unresectable or metastatic

M. Tetsuhito · Y. Komatsu (✉)
Cancer Center, Hokkaido University Hospital, Hokkaido, Japan
e-mail: muranaka@frontier.hokudai.ac.jp; ykomatsu@ac.cyberhome.ne.jp

Y. Kurokawa, Y. Komatsu (eds.), *Gastrointestinal Stromal Tumor*,
https://doi.org/10.1007/978-981-13-3206-7_6

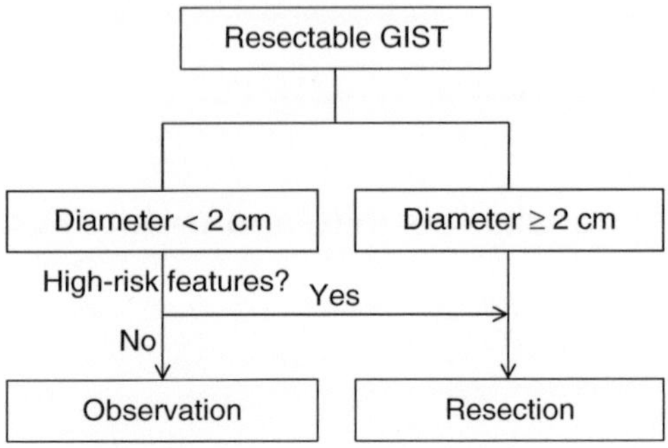

Fig. 6.1 Strategy for resectable gastrointestinal stromal tumors

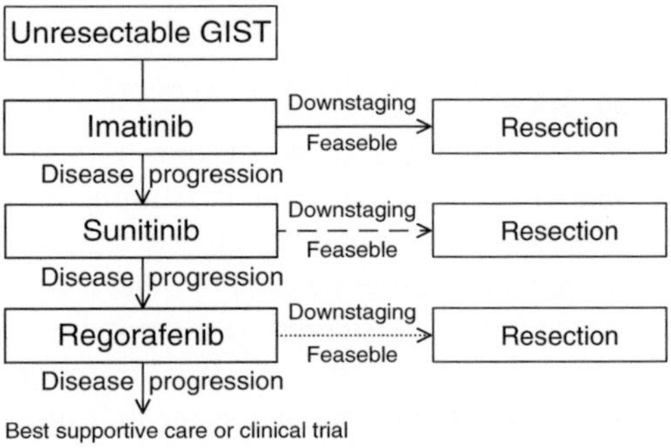

Fig. 6.2 Strategy for unresectable gastrointestinal stromal tumors

GISTs. Prior to therapy initiation, GISTs should be evaluated using computed tomography (CT) and/or magnetic resonance imaging (MRI), pathological tests, and gene mutation analysis. For very small gastric GISTs, abdominal/pelvic CT and/or MRI should be performed. For all other GISTs, chest, abdominal, and pelvic CT and/or abdominal/pelvic MRI should be performed. As GISTs sometimes metastasize to bones, positron emission tomography (PET) or bone scintigraphy should be performed when pathological fractures, bone pain, or increases in alkaline phosphatase levels are noted (Figs. 6.1 and 6.2).

6.2 Very Small GISTs (<2 cm)

Very small GISTs can be incidentally found as sub-mucosal tumors using endoscopy or CT. After identification, pathological diagnosis should be performed using endoscopic ultrasound-guided fine-needle aspiration (EUS-FNA) [2]. When very small GISTs do not have any high-risk EUS features, including irregular borders, cystic spaces, ulceration, echogenic foci, and heterogeneity, periodic radiographic surveillance is recommended. EUS surveillance should be considered only after a thorough discussion with the patient regarding the risks and benefits of EUS [3]. When very small GISTs have high-risk EUS features, complete surgical resection is recommended. After resection, periodic surveillance is recommended if the risk of recurrence is low (see Tables 6.1, 6.2, and 6.3). However, if the risk of recurrence is

Table 6.1 Risk classification (Fletcher et al. [4])

Classification	Size	Mitotic count
Very low risk	<2 cm	<5/50 HPFs
Low risk	2–5 cm	<5/50 HPFs
Intermediate risk	<5 cm	6–10/50 HPFs
	5–10 cm	<5/50 HPFs
High risk	>5 cm	>5/50 HPFs
	>10 cm	Any mitotic rate
	Any size	>10/50 HPFs

HPF high power field, ×400 magnification

Table 6.2 Risk classification (Miettinen and Lasota [5])

Mitotic index	Size (cm)	Stomach	Small intestine	Duodenum	Colon and rectum
≤5/50 HPFs	≤2	None	None	None	None
≤5/50 HPFs	2< and ≤5	Very low	Low	Low	Low
≤5/50 HPFs	5< and ≤10	Low	Moderate	Insuff. data	Insuff. data
≤5/50 HPFs	10≤	Moderate	High	High	High
>5/50 HPFs	≤2	None	High	None	High
>5/50 HPFs	2< and ≤5	Moderate	High	High	High
>5/50 HPFs	5< and ≤10	High	High	Insuff. data	Insuff. data
>5/50 HPFs	10≤	High	High	High	High

HPF high power field, ×400 magnification

Table 6.3 Risk classification (Joensuu [6] and Rutkowski et al. [7])

Risk category	Tumor size in largest dimension (cm)	Mitotic index (per 50 HPFs)	Primary tumor site
Very low risk	<2.0	≤5	Any
Low risk	2.1–5.0	≤5	Any
Intermediate risk	2.1–5.0	>5	Gastric
	<5.0	6–10	Any
	5.1–10.0	≤5	Gastric
High risk	Any	Any	Tumor rupture
	>10 cm	Any	Any
	Any	>10	Any
	>5.0	>5	Any
	2.1–5.0	>5	Nongastric
	5.1–10.0	≤5	Nongastric

HPF high power field, ×400 magnification

significant, postoperative imatinib administration for at least 36 months should be considered, according to the results of a randomized trial (SSGXVIII/AIO) showing that relapse-free survival and overall survival were better with postoperative imatinib administration for 36 months than for that for 12 months in patients with a high estimated risk of recurrence (tumor size >5 cm with a high mitotic rate, tumor rupture, or risk of recurrence greater than 50% after surgery) [8]. In addition, the approach of periodic surveillance every 6–12 months for 5 years followed by annual imaging is recommended.

6.3 Localized Resectable GISTs (Initially Resectable)

Resection should be considered in all localized resectable GISTs when preoperative imatinib administration is not indicated. Lymph node dissection is usually not required because of the low incidence of nodal metastasis in cases of GISTs, except succinate dehydrogenase (SDH)-deficient GISTs, which often occur in patients with Carney–Stratakis syndrome or Carney triad. Laparoscopic resection can be considered for GISTs at appropriate anatomical locations. Surgeons need to pay close attention to avoid damaging the frail pseudocapsule of the GIST. Complete resection is the only curative treatment for these GISTs, and preoperative imatinib administration may make it difficult to accurately assess the recurrence risk after surgery. It is necessary to assess the recurrence risk through pathological findings, including anatomical location, tumor size, and mitotic rate in the most proliferative area of the GIST [5–7].

Even if the tumor is completely resected, postoperative imatinib administration for at least 36 months should be considered in patients with a significant risk of recurrence (intermediate or high risk), according to the findings of the SSGXVIII/AIO trial [8]. Additionally, the ACOSOG trial Z9001 suggested that postoperative imatinib administration improved relapse-free survival in patients with GISTs ≥3 cm in size showing a significant risk of recurrence (intermediate or high risk) [9]. Moreover, the approach of periodic surveillance every 3–6 months for 5 years followed by annual imaging is recommended.

If complete resection is achieved and the risk of recurrence is low, adjuvant imatinib should not be considered because of the lack of evidence. In such cases, history taking and physical examination should be performed every 3–6 months for 5 years followed by annual imaging.

When a persistent gross residual GIST is identified after surgery, imatinib administration should be strongly considered until no evidence of the disease, occurrence of intolerable adverse events, or progression of the disease. Repeat resection is generally not indicated in cases showing microscopically positive margins on final pathological assessment.

No randomized controlled phase III trial has confirmed the benefits of neoadjuvant imatinib for locally advanced GISTs; thus, preoperative imatinib should be considered only if surgical morbidity can be reduced by down-staging the tumor preoperatively. Imatinib administration may require 6 months or more for maximal response.

Gene mutation analysis is recommended prior to neoadjuvant imatinib administration to predict imatinib efficacy. Approximately 90% of GISTs with *KIT* exon 11 mutation tend to respond to imatinib therapy, whereas about 50% of GISTs with *KIT* exon 9 mutation respond to 400-mg imatinib, and the response might improve with the use of 800-mg imatinib. Almost all GISTs with *PDGFRA* gene mutation, except D842V, respond to imatinib. GISTs that show SDH deficiency and *NF1* or *BRAF* mutation do not appropriately respond to imatinib. For GISTs that show SDH deficiency, sunitinib administration should be considered. Wild-type GISTs that do not show any gene mutations have a 0–45% likelihood of responding to imatinib [10–13].

6.4 Locally Advanced GISTs (Initially Unresectable)

Resection should be initially considered for localized GISTs. However, locally advanced GISTs can sometimes be difficult to resect with acceptable surgical morbidity because of direct invasion to other organs or inappropriate locations for resection. Neoadjuvant imatinib can be considered when surgical morbidity can be reduced or when initial complete resection is not possible [14, 15]. As mentioned earlier, imatinib administration for 6 months or more might be required. Gene mutation analysis is recommended prior to neoadjuvant imatinib administration. Approximately 90% of GISTs with *KIT* exon 11 mutation tend to respond to imatinib therapy, whereas about 50% of GISTs with *KIT* exon 9 mutation respond to 400-mg imatinib, and the response might improve with the use of 800-mg imatinib. Almost all GISTs with *PDGFRA* gene mutation, except D842V, respond to imatinib. GISTs that show SDH deficiency and *NF1* or *BRAF* mutation do not appropriately respond to imatinib. For GISTs that show SDH deficiency, sunitinib administration should be considered. Wild-type GISTs that do not show any gene mutations have a 0–45% likelihood of responding to imatinib [10–13]. PET can help in the assessment of imatinib activity after 2–4 weeks of therapy [16]. Imatinib administration can be continued until just before surgery and restarted as soon as possible after surgery when the patient is able to receive oral medications. Sunitinib or regorafenib need to be discontinued at least 1 week prior to surgery.

Close monitoring is needed because GISTs sometimes grow rapidly. When severe adverse events occur with imatinib, which cannot be managed even with maximum supportive care, sunitinib administration should be considered. Surgery should be considered if GISTs show active bleeding or severe symptoms.

Continuation of imatinib administration should be considered after complete resection if therapy is effective preoperatively. No randomized trials have mentioned the duration of postoperative imatinib in these patients.

6.5 Unresectable or Metastatic GISTs

6.5.1 Initial Approach for Unresectable or Metastatic GISTs

When GISTs are believed to be unresectable on abdominal/pelvic CT and/or MRI and are pathologically confirmed, surgery cannot be initially considered. GISTs sometimes metastasize to the lungs, skin, and bones, and additional chest radiography/CT or PET can be considered prior to imatinib administration [17]. Imatinib at 400 mg a day is strongly recommended as the first-line treatment in patients with unresectable or metastatic GISTs [18]. Gene mutation analysis is recommended prior to neoadjuvant imatinib administration. Approximately 90% of GISTs with *KIT* exon 11 mutation tend to respond to imatinib therapy, whereas about 50% of GISTs with *KIT* exon 9 mutation respond to 400-mg imatinib, and the response might improve with the use of 800-mg imatinib. Almost all GISTs with *PDGFRA* gene mutation, except D842V, respond to imatinib. GISTs that show SDH deficiency and *NF1* or *BRAF* mutation do not appropriately respond to imatinib. For GISTs that show SDH deficiency, sunitinib administration should be considered. Wild-type GISTs that do not show any gene mutations have a 0–45% likelihood of responding to imatinib [10–13]. PET can help in the assessment of imatinib activity after 2–4 weeks of therapy [16]. Response assessment using abdominal/pelvic CT or MRI might be needed every 8–12 weeks. PET may be useful to determine disease progression if CT/MRI findings are ambiguous. If treatment is successful, the frequency of imaging can be decreased. The possibility of surgery should be considered during the treatment course of imatinib. Imatinib should be continued if resection is not feasible and an intolerable adverse event has not occurred.

6.5.2 Second-Line Treatment for Unresectable or Metastatic GISTs

If disease progression is noted on CT/MRI, it is recommended to use sunitinib instead of imatinib, unless patient adherence is poor. Unresectable or metastatic GISTs with acquired resistance are usually associated with a secondary mutation in *KIT* or *PDGFRA*. SDH-deficient GISTs usually have a better likelihood of responding to sunitinib [19]. A placebo-controlled randomized controlled trial showed that sunitinib improved progression-free survival (27.3 weeks in the sunitinib group vs. 6.4 weeks in the placebo group; hazard ratio 0.33; $p < 0.0001$) [20]. Sunitinib is administered orally once daily at a starting dose of 50 mg in a 6-week cycle with 4 weeks on and 2 weeks off treatment, and the dose is appropriately reduced to 37.5 mg or 25 mg a day when severe adverse events occur. The most common treatment-related adverse events are fatigue, diarrhea, skin discoloration, and nausea, but severe myelosuppression sometimes occurs. It should be noted that the duration of myelosuppression might be longer with sunitinib than with other anti-cancer chemotherapy drugs. Response assessment using abdominal/pelvic CT or MRI might be needed every 8–12 weeks. Unresectable or metastatic GISTs with acquired resistance usually cause the secondary gene mutation in *KIT* or *PDGFRA*. SDH-deficient GIST usually has a better likelihood of response to sunitinib [20].

6.5.3 Third-Line Treatment for Unresectable or Metastatic GISTs

The GRID trial, a placebo-controlled randomized phase III trial, showed that regorafenib administration in patients with unresectable or metastatic GISTs, who showed previous imatinib or sunitinib failure, resulted in an improvement in progression-free survival (4.8 months in the regorafenib group vs. 0.9 months in the placebo group; hazard ratio 0.27; $p < 0.0001$) [21]. Oral regorafenib was administered at 160 mg a day for the first 3 weeks in a 4-week cycle. As this trial allowed placebo crossover to regorafenib, the benefit of regorafenib with regard to overall survival was not assessed. The most common regorafenib-related adverse events of grade 3 or higher were hypertension, hand–foot skin reaction, and diarrhea. Life-threatening liver injury may rarely occur, and liver function should be assessed every week for 8 weeks from the first regorafenib administration. We should note that these evidences must be applied to ECOG performance status 0 or 1. Life-long continuation of regorafenib therapy should be considered for palliation of symptoms as part of best supportive care. Regorafenib is the last drug option, and thus, patients should be strongly encouraged to participate in clinical trials.

6.5.4 Other Optional Treatments

Some trials have supported the benefits of optional treatments, but no randomized phase III trial has confirmed benefits with regard to patient survival.

Hasegawa et al. reported on patients who had focal lesions associated with secondary resistant GISTs during imatinib treatment and who underwent surgical interventions, such as resection, radiofrequency ablation, and their combination. The median time to progression was 5.5 months [22]. Although the findings supported these treatments, there is no randomized phase III trial on these treatments. Further clinical trials are warranted.

Kobayashi et al. reported the efficacy of hepatic artery chemoembolization in a single-arm trial [23]. They evaluated 85 of 110 patients with GISTs who underwent hepatic artery chemoembolization, and reported that 14% of the patients had partial response and 74% had stable disease. The median progression-free survival was 8.2 months. Cao et al. reported that transcatheter arterial chemoembolization achieved partial response in 12 of 22 patients [24]. Additionally, Rathmann et al. reported the benefits of radioembolization in patients with GIST-associated liver metastases [25]. As these trials are single-arm studies or small studies, further clinical trials are warranted.

References

1. National Comprehensive Cancer Network Guidelines. https://www.nccn.org/professionals/physician_gls/. Accessed 8 Sept 2018.
2. Sepe PS, Brugge WR. A guide for the diagnosis and management of gastrointestinal stromal cell tumors. Nat Rev Gastroenterol Hepatol. 2009;6(6):363–71.
3. ASGE Standards of Practice Committee, Evans JA, Chandrasekhara V, Chathadi KV, Decker GA, Early DS, Fisher DA, Foley K, Hwang JH, Jue TL, Lightdale JR, Pasha SF, Sharaf R, Shergill AK, Cash BD, JM DW. The role of endoscopy in the management of premalignant and malignant conditions of the stomach. Gastrointest Endosc. 2015;82(1):1–8.
4. Fletcher CD, Berman JJ, Corless C, Gorstein F, Lasota J, Longley BJ, Miettinen M, O'Leary TJ, Remotti H, Rubin BP, Shmookler B, Sobin LH, Weiss SW. Diagnosis of gastrointestinal stromal tumors: a consensus approach. Hum Pathol. 2002;33(5):459–65.
5. Miettinen M, Lasota J. Gastrointestinal stromal tumors: pathology and prognosis at different sites. Semin Diagn Pathol. 2006;23(2):70–83.
6. Joensuu H. Risk stratification of patients diagnosed with gastrointestinal stromal tumor. Hum Pathol. 2008;39(10):1411–9.

7. Rutkowski P, Bylina E, Wozniak A, Nowecki ZI, Osuch C, Matlok M, Switaj T, Michej W, Wroński M, Głuszek S, Kroc J, Nasierowska-Guttmejer A, Joensuu H. Validation of the Joensuu risk criteria for primary resectable gastrointestinal stromal tumour – the impact of tumour rupture on patient outcomes. Eur J Surg Oncol. 2011;37(10):890–6.
8. Eisenberg BL. The SSG XVIII/AIO trial: results change the current adjuvant treatment recommendations for gastrointestinal stromal tumors. Am J Clin Oncol. 2013;36(1):89–90.
9. Corless CL, Ballman KV, Antonescu CR, Kolesnikova V, Maki RG, Pisters PW, Blackstein ME, Blanke CD, Demetri GD, Heinrich MC, von Mehren M, Patel S, McCarter MD, Owzar K, DeMatteo RP. Pathologic and molecular features correlate with long-term outcome after adjuvant therapy of resected primary GI stromal tumor: the ACOSOG Z9001 trial. J Clin Oncol. 2014;32(15):1563–70.
10. Rossi S, Gasparotto D, Miceli R, Toffolatti L, Gallina G, Scaramel E, Marzotto A, Boscato E, Messerini L, Bearzi I, Mazzoleni G, Capella C, Arrigoni G, Sonzogni A, Sidoni A, Mariani L, Amore P, Gronchi A, Casali PG, Maestro R, Dei Tos AP. KIT, PDGFRA, and BRAF mutational spectrum impacts on the natural history of imatinib-naive localized GIST: a population-based study. Am J Surg Pathol. 2015;39(7):922–30.
11. Ahmad F, Lad P, Bhatia S, Das BR. Molecular spectrum of c-KIT and PDGFRA gene mutations in gastro intestinal stromal tumor: determination of frequency, distribution pattern and identification of novel mutations in Indian patients. Med Oncol. 2015;32(1):424.
12. Miettinen M, Sobin LH, Lasota J. Gastrointestinal stromal tumors of the stomach: a clinicopathologic, immunohistochemical, and molecular genetic study of 1765 cases with long-term follow-up. Am J Surg Pathol. 2005;29(1):52–68.
13. Kumari N, Priyaa V, Shukla P, Kumar A, Aggarwal R, Krishnani N. Gastrointestinal stromal tumor: genotype frequency and prognostic relevance. Appl Immunohistochem Mol Morphol. 2018;26(3):153–60.
14. Xu J, Ling TL, Wang M, Zhao WY, Cao H. Preoperative imatinib treatment in patients with advanced gastrointestinal stromal tumors: patient experiences and systematic review of 563 patients. Int Surg. 2015;100(5):860–9.
15. Rutkowski P, Gronchi A, Hohenberger P, Bonvalot S, Schöffski P, Bauer S, Fumagalli E, Nyckowski P, Nguyen BP, Kerst JM, Fiore M, Bylina E, Hoiczyk M, Cats A, Casali PG, Le Cesne A, Treckmann J, Stoeckle E, de Wilt JH, Sleijfer S, Tielen R, van der Graaf W, Verhoef C, van Coevorden F. Neoadjuvant imatinib in locally advanced gastrointestinal stromal tumors (GIST): the EORTC STBSG experience. Ann Surg Oncol. 2013;20(9):2937–43.
16. McAuliffe JC, Hunt KK, Lazar AJ, Choi H, Qiao W, Thall P, Pollock RE, Benjamin RS, Trent JC. A randomized, phase II study of preoperative plus postoperative imatinib in GIST: evidence of rapid radiographic response and temporal induction of tumor cell apoptosis. Ann Surg Oncol. 2009;16(4):910–9.
17. Dematteo RP, Heinrich MC, El-Rifai WM, Demetri G. Clinical management of gastrointestinal stromal tumors: before and after STI-571. Hum Pathol. 2002;33(5):466–77.
18. Verweij J, Casali PG, Zalcberg J, LeCesne A, Reichardt P, Blay JY, Issels R, van Oosterom A, Hogendoorn PC, Van Glabbeke M, Bertulli R, Judson I. Progression-free survival in gastrointestinal stromal tumours with high-dose imatinib: randomised trial. Lancet. 2004;364(9440):1127–34.
19. Ben-Ami E, Barysauskas CM, von Mehren M, Heinrich MC, Corless CL, Butrynski JE, Morgan JA, Wagner AJ, Choy E, Yap JT, Van den Abbeele AD, Solomon SM, Fletcher JA, Demetri GD, George S. Long-term follow-up results of the multicenter phase II trial of regorafenib in patients with metastatic and/or unresectable GI stromal tumor after failure of standard tyrosine kinase inhibitor therapy. Ann Oncol. 2016;27(9):1794–9.
20. Demetri GD, van Oosterom AT, Garrett CR, Blackstein ME, Shah MH, Verweij J, McArthur G, Judson IR, Heinrich MC, Morgan JA, Desai J, Fletcher CD, George S, Bello CL, Huang X, Baum CM, Casali PG. Efficacy and safety of sunitinib in patients with advanced gastrointestinal stromal tumour after failure of imatinib: a randomised controlled trial. Lancet. 2006;368(9544):1329–38.

21. Demetri GD, Reichardt P, Kang YK, Blay JY, Rutkowski P, Gelderblom H, Hohenberger P, Leahy M, von Mehren M, Joensuu H, Badalamenti G, Blackstein M, Le Cesne A, Schöffski P, Maki RG, Bauer S, Nguyen BB, Xu J, Nishida T, Chung J, Kappeler C, Kuss I, Laurent D, Casali PG, study investigators GRID. Efficacy and safety of regorafenib for advanced gastrointestinal stromal tumours after failure of imatinib and sunitinib (GRID): an international, multicentre, randomised, placebo-controlled, phase 3 trial. Lancet. 2013;381(9863):295–302.
22. Hasegawa J, Kanda T, Hirota S, Fukuda M, Nishitani A, Takahashi T, Kurosaki I, Tsutsui S, Hatakeyama K, Nishida T. Surgical interventions for focal progression of advanced gastrointestinal stromal tumors during imatinib therapy. Int J Clin Oncol. 2007;12(3):212–7.
23. Kobayashi K, Gupta S, Trent JC, Vauthey JN, Krishnamurthy S, Ensor J, Ahrar K, Wallace MJ, Madoff DC, Murthy R, McRae SE, Hicks ME. Hepatic artery chemoembolization for 110 gastrointestinal stromal tumors: response, survival, and prognostic factors. Cancer. 2006;107(12):2833–41.
24. Cao G, Li J, Shen L, Zhu X. Transcatheter arterial chemoembolization for gastrointestinal stromal tumors with liver metastases. World J Gastroenterol. 2012;18(42):6134–40.
25. Rathmann N, Diehl SJ, Dinter D, Schütte J, Pink D, Schoenberg SO, Hohenberger P. Radioembolization in patients with progressive gastrointestinal stromal tumor liver metastases undergoing treatment with tyrosine kinase inhibitors. J Vasc Interv Radiol. 2015;26(2):231–8.

Surgery

7

Souya Nunobe

Abstract

The number 1 option for gastrointestinal stromal tumor (GIST) treatment is surgery. Given an organ-sparing approach, it is critical to completely remove the tumor without damaging the pseudocapsule. Removal of the lymph nodes is usually not necessary.

Normally a laparoscopic excision is used on lesions under 5 cm. When using the magnification from a laparoscope, the blood vessels that are manipulated are held to a minimum and the nerves can be preserved as much as possible. This approach has provided good post-operative gastric peristaltic movement. In recent years, a laparoscopic endoscopic cooperative surgery (LECS), which uses both a laparoscope and an endoscope, has been performed in order to prevent excessive resection of the healthy gastric wall. By minimizing the resection of the gastric wall particularly for a GIST that is located at the esophagogastric junction, the cardia can be spared and a proximal gastrectomy can be avoided. The application of LECS was used on lesions that did not include any mucosal lesions since the gastric wall was opened. However, it also became possible to perform a resection on GISTs with ulcerated lesions without scattering tumor cells inside the abdominal cavity by using LECS related techniques, such as an inverted LECS. It is important in terms of oncology to grab the tumor directly and avoid contact with organs inside the abdominal cavity with mucosal lesions.

A post-operative follow-up is performed depending on the risk category assigned by the National Institutes of Health (NIH). For high risk or clinically malignant GIST cases, a CT scan follow-up is appropriate for the first 3 years once every 4–6 months, and then once a year until the 10th year after surgery.

S. Nunobe (✉)
Department of Gastroenterological Surgery, Cancer Institute Ariake Hospital, Tokyo, Japan
e-mail: souya.nunobe@jfcr.or.jp

Y. Kurokawa, Y. Komatsu (eds.), *Gastrointestinal Stromal Tumor*,
https://doi.org/10.1007/978-981-13-3206-7_7

Keywords
GIST · Laparoscopic local excision · Laparoscopic endoscopic cooperative surgery (LECS)

7.1 Principle of the Surgical Treatment

The number 1 option for resectable primary GIST treatment is surgery [1, 2]. As a general rule for surgical treatment, the priority order is as follows: (1) Complete resection. (2) Maintain safe margins for surgery without damaging the pseudocapsule, leaving a gross stump that tests negative. (3) Partial resection with an organ-sparing approach is recommended. (4) Preventive and systematic removal of the lymph nodes is not necessary [3].

When a GIST with tumor progression has severely adhered or invaded the neighboring organ, an en bloc resection with the tumor should be performed when possible in order to prevent damaging the pseudocapsule, scattering of tumor cells inside the abdominal cavity, or causing their outflow, which can be characteristic when performing a difficult or forced ablation of the affected organ.

In addition, when imatinib is used for treatment prior to surgery, a histopathological examination is required to confirm the tumor as a GIST as well as imatinib's efficacy at the GIST's early stage of approximately 1 month [4, 5].

7.2 Indication of Surgery

We would like you to refer to the treatment algorithm in the previous section for surgical indication. Surgery, including relative indication, is usually used on gastric submucosal tumors (SMTs) that are a minimum of 2 cm. There are many facilities that use laparoscopic local excision (LALE) for GISTs that are less than 5 cm. An open abdominal surgery is often used for GISTs that are a minimum of 5 cm because it is difficult to handle the tumors using forceps.

There are three major types of GIST forms: luminal, intramural, and extramural growth types. LALE is a good application for extramural growth tumors. Laparoscopic endoscopic cooperative surgery (LECS), which uses both a laparoscope and an endoscope, has been devised for tumors, such as luminal and intramural growth types, as well as tumors close to the cardia and pylorus [6–8]. The LECS technique offers a tremendous advantage because it can minimize gastric deformity after the tumor excision, and stereotypical surgeries, such as a proximal gastrectomy, can also be avoided for tumors that are close to the cardia, etc.

7.3 Laparoscopic Local Excision (LALE)

7.3.1 Setup for Laparoscopic Surgery

The patients were placed in the lithotomy position under general anesthesia. The operator stood at the right side of the patient, the first assistant stood at the left side of the patient, and the laparoscopist stood between the patients' legs.

A camera port was inserted via a 12-mm port in the umbilicus, using an open technique. Four additional ports (three 5-mm ports and one 12-mm port) were inserted into the left upper, left lower, right upper, and right lower quadrants, respectively, under pneumoperitoneum (10 mmHg) (Fig. 7.1). A 12-mm port was additionally used when the manipulation of the stapling devices was limited by the location of the tumor, such as in the esophagogastric junction.

The surgery method performed uses a single incision or reduced port surgery depending on the facility; however, this surgery method proved difficult in some instances due to the position of the tumor, and additional measures such as additional ports are incorporated.

7.3.2 Resection of the Tumor During LALE

For lesions where LALE is applied, there are many cases in which the lesion position is clear only when observing using a normal laparoscopy. Using the

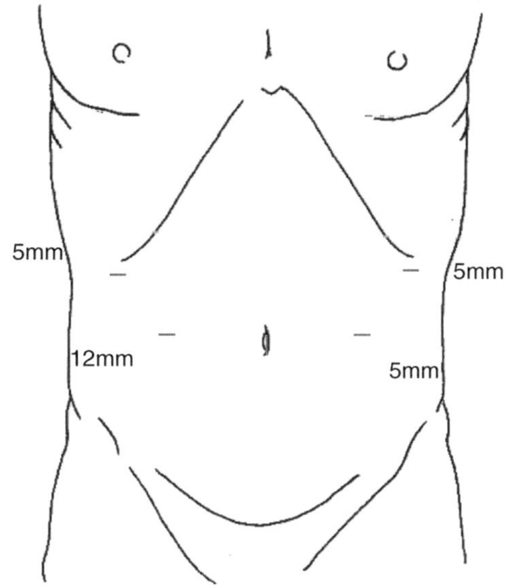

Fig. 7.1 Port placement. A camera port is inserted via a 12-mm port in the umbilicus, using an open technique. Four additional ports (three 5-mm ports and one 12-mm port) are inserted into the left upper, left lower, right upper, and right lower quadrants, respectively

magnification on the laparoscope can help minimize the surrounding blood vessels that are manipulated. If the lesion is on the lesser curvature of the stomach, an approach is taken to minimize manipulation of blood vessels as close to the gastric wall as possible, so as to spare the anterior vagal trunk when manipulating the blood vessels. It is said that many patients experience gastric stasis after surgery for local excisions of lesions on the lesser curvature. If steps can be taken to ensure the preservation of nerves, then the good post-operative gastric peristalsis can be maintained. In addition, for small lesions on the lesser curvature that exist inside the gastropancreatic ligament, tumors can be looked like luminal growth type prior to surgery (Fig. 7.2). Nonetheless, there are some lesions where blood vessels are first manipulated and then discovered to be extramural growth tumors. Furthermore, there are cases in which it is difficult to distinguish whether the lesions on the posterior wall are closer to the greater curvature or to the lesser curvature prior to surgery (Fig. 7.3). We have also discovered that there are cases in which the posterior

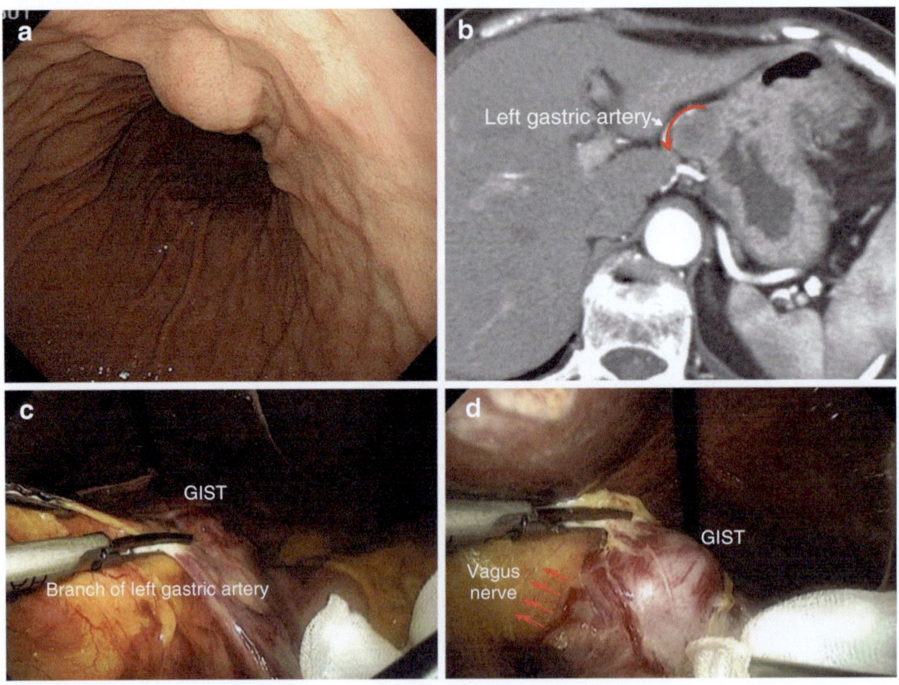

Fig. 7.2 Dissection around submucosal tumor on the lesser curvature at the middle stomach. For small lesions on the lesser curvature that exist inside the gastropancreatic ligament, tumors can be looked like luminal growth type prior to surgery by endoscopic finding (**a**). Actually, tumor is extraluminal growth type after dissection around the tumor (**d**). If steps can be taken to ensure the preservation of nerves (**b**: red arrow, **d**), then the good post-operative gastric peristalsis can be maintained. Dissection line showed by red arrow is inside of the left gastric artery for preservation of vagus nerve (**c**)

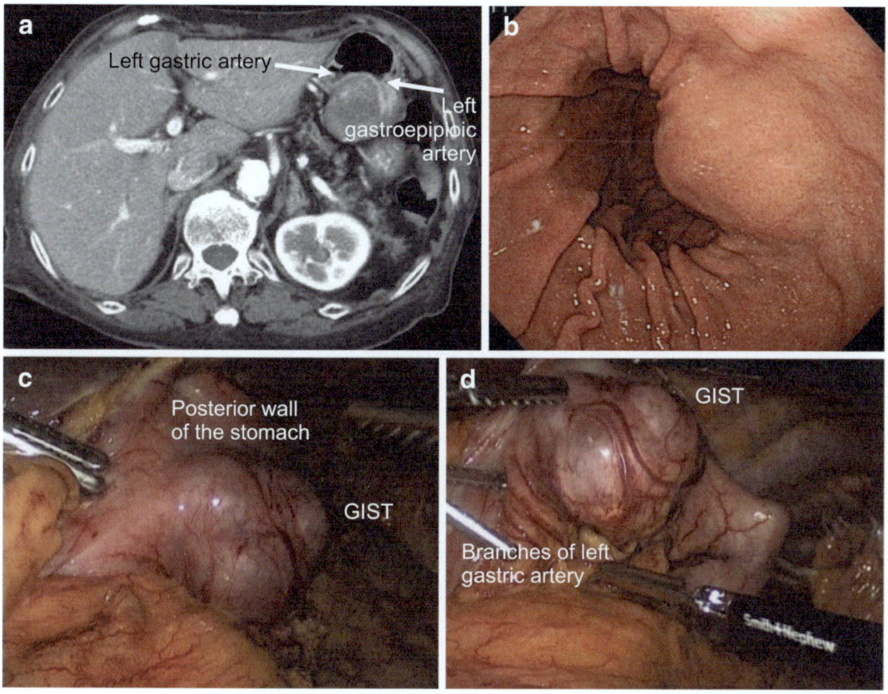

Fig. 7.3 A case in which it is difficult to distinguish whether the lesions on the posterior wall are closer to the greater curvature or to the lesser curvature prior to surgery. (**a**) CT finding shows that the tumor is located on the posterior wall between left gastric artery and left gastroepiploic artery. (**b**) Endoscopic finding shows the tumor located on the posterior wall. (**c**, **d**) Actually, tumor located on the posterior wall near the branches of left gastric artery

wall lesion was thought to be close to the greater curvature, but after manipulating the blood vessels on the greater curvature and looking carefully with the lesser sac opened, the lesion was actually close to the lesser curvature. Ultimately, the blood vessels on the lesser curvature are manipulated, and the complication of the sutures failing due to poor blood flow could occur. As a result, the position of the lesion is not easy to diagnosis merely with an examination prior to surgery. It is essential to observe carefully during the operation and to thoroughly check the surrounding blood vessels that should be manipulated.

After the blood vessels are manipulated, a resection is performed on a tumor where a stapler is used. For lesions closer to the greater curvature, the resection may be easier when there are few or no complications, such as the direction of the resection and the range of the resection on the gastric wall. For lesions on the lesser curvature, resecting along the longitudinal axis can help prevent poor peristalsis when the stomach becomes shaped like a dumbbell after the resection (Fig. 7.4). Finally, the staple line should be carefully checked. If staples do not form a complete seal for the repair, interrupted sutures should be added to strengthen the repair.

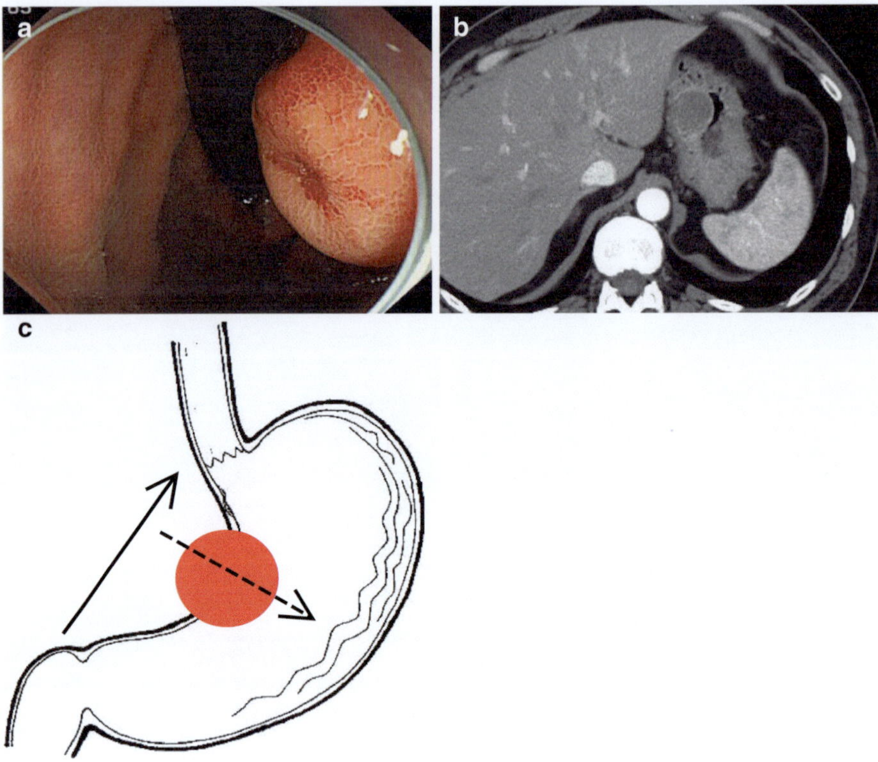

Fig. 7.4 Resection for tumor located at the lesser curvature. Endoscopic finding and CT show tumor is located on the lesser curvature in the middle stomach (**a**, **b**). For lesions on the lesser curvature, resecting along the longitudinal axis can help prevent poor peristalsis when the stomach becomes shaped like a dumbbell after the resection (**c**)

7.4 Laparoscopic Endoscopic Cooperative Surgery (LECS) [6, 7]

To facilitate appropriate resection, we developed a laparoscopic endoscopic cooperative surgery (LECS) technique that combines laparoscopic gastric resection with endoscopic submucosal dissection (ESD), and we have used this procedure to resect gastric SMTs. In this procedure, the tumor location and an appropriate resection line are confirmed endoscopically, and followed by submucosal dissection using intraluminal endoscopy. The seromuscular layer is then dissected laparoscopically, and the incision line is closed using a laparoscopic stapling device. We have got the good results after LECS for the gastric SMT and the original procedure was named "classical LECS" [9].

Many researchers have reported that classical LECS is a feasible and safe surgical procedure for the treatment of gastric SMTs [7, 8, 10–12]. The benefit of classical LECS is the completeness of the resection with a minimal margin. Classical LECS is technically easier than the modified LECS procedures. Thus, classical

LECS can be applied to any tumor location including the esophagogastric junction. We can make the best use of the advantages of LECS for gastric SMTs located at the esophagogastric junction by avoiding conventional total gastrectomy or proximal gastrectomy. Hoteya et al. reported the feasibility of classical LECS for gastric SMTs located at the esophagogastric junction [12].

A limitation of classical LECS is the possibility of tumor and gastric juice contamination into the abdominal cavity due to opening of the gastric wall during the procedure. Accordingly, classical LECS can be applied to gastric SMTs without a mucosal lesion.

7.4.1 Indication for Classical LECS and Inverted LECS

We first applied LECS to gastric SMTs without ulcerative lesions because we worried that tumor cells would seed into the peritoneal cavity; the procedure was named "classical LECS." The maximum tumor size was limited to a diameter of 50 mm, regardless of the location, according to the indications for laparoscopic resection of GISTs. Recently, we have applied LECS to SMTs with ulcerative lesions and early gastric cancer that would have been difficult to treat using ESD because of scarring or broad lateral spreading; the procedure was named "Inverted LECS" [13].

7.4.2 Setup for LECS

Setup for LECS is such as LALE for laparoscopic procedure. Additionally, the endoscopic operator and the assistant were positioned at the patient's head.

7.4.3 Confirmation of Tumor Location and Blood Vessel Preparation

The tumor location was confirmed via intraluminal endoscopy during surgery (H260; Olympus, Tokyo, Japan). Biopsy forceps were used to exert pressure on the mucosal side of the stomach wall to confirm the location of the tumor on the laparoscopic image. The blood vessels in the excision area were prepared using an ultrasonically activated device (Harmonic Ultrasonic Scalpel; Ethicon Endo-Surgery, Cincinnati, Ohio). We recommend that the area of blood vessels manipulation be minimized to prevent post-operative gastric stasis.

7.4.4 Endoscopic Submucosal Resection Around the Tumor and Laparoscopic Seromuscular Dissection (Figs. 7.5 and 7.6)

The periphery of the tumor was carefully marked using a standard needle-knife with a forced 20-W coagulation current (ESG-100; Olympus, Tokyo, Japan) as close as

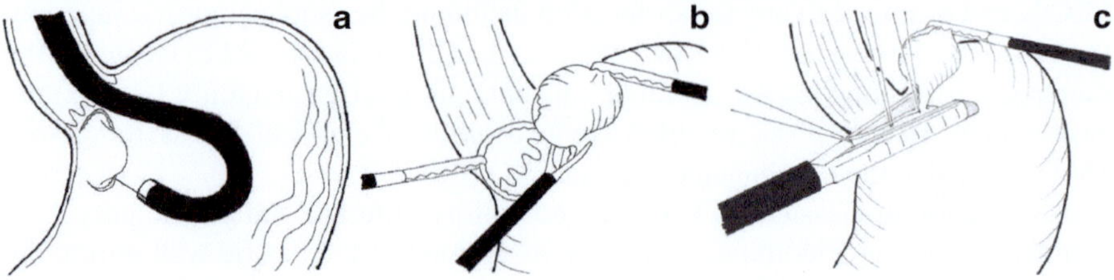

Fig. 7.5 Laparoscopic endoscopic cooperative surgery (LECS) for the gastric GIST. (**a**) After injection of 10% glycerin into the submucosal layer, a small initial incision is made using a standard needle-knife in the 100-W Endo-Cut mode, and the tip of an IT-2 knife is inserted into the submucosal layer for dissection around the tumor. The marked area is then cut circumferentially, using the IT-2 knife. (**b**) The full-thickness incision is performed laparoscopically or endoscopically with laparoscopic assistance as far as possible, and the remaining part of the full-thickness wall dissection is usually performed laparoscopically. (**c**) After the tumor has been resected, the edge of the incision line is temporarily closed using hand-sewn sutures. The incision line is then closed using a laparoscopic stapling device

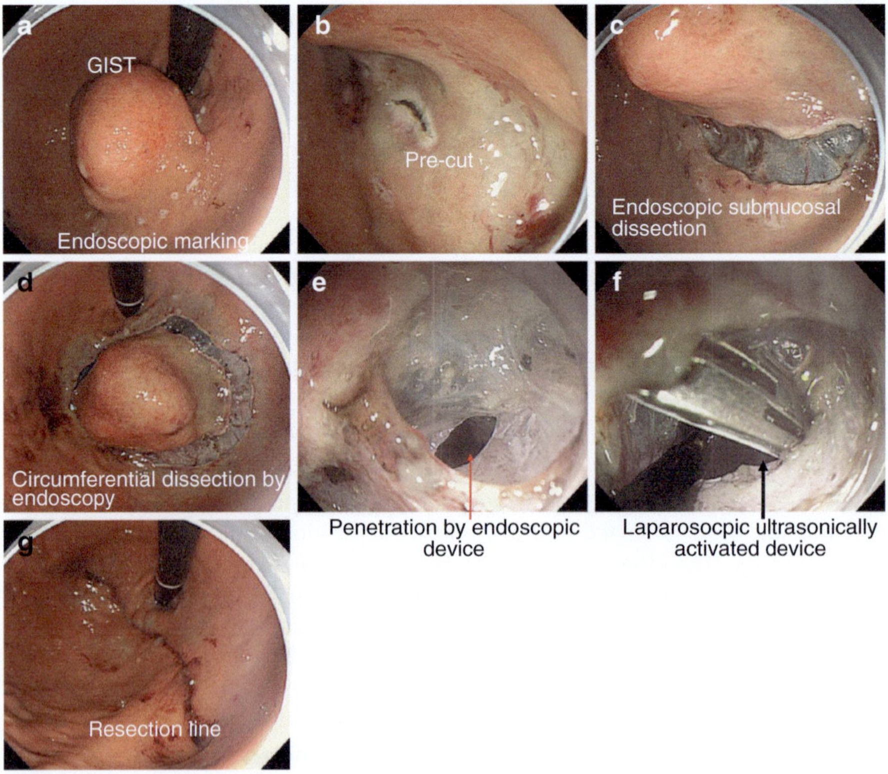

Fig. 7.6 Endoscopic findings during LECS procedure. (**a**) Endoscopic marking around the tumor. (**b**) Pre-cut. (**c**) Endoscopic submucosal dissection by IT-knife. (**d**) Circumferential dissection by endoscopy. (**e**) Penetration of the gastric wall by endoscopic device. (**f**) Confirmation of the laparoscopic ultrasonically activated device by intra-gastric endoscope. (**g**) Tumor is resected by LECS procedure with less deformation of the gastric body

possible to the tumor edge. After injection of 10% glycerin into the submucosal layer, a small initial incision was made using a standard needle-knife in the 100-W Endo-Cut mode, and the tip of an IT-2 knife (KD-611L; Olympus, Tokyo, Japan) was inserted into the submucosal layer. The marked area was then cut circumferentially, using the IT-2 knife in the 100-W Endo-Cut mode. The opening of the submucosa was then pushed toward the serosa using a standard needle-knife. The tip of the standard needle-knife, which could be seen on the laparoscopic image (beyond the seromuscular layer), was used to perforate the seromuscular layer. The tip of the IT-2 knife was inserted into the perforation, and seromuscular dissection was initiated along the incision line of the submucosal layer. The full-thickness incision was performed endoscopically with laparoscopic assistance as far as possible, and the remaining part of the full-thickness wall dissection was performed laparoscopically.

After the tumor had been resected, the edge of the incision line was temporarily closed using hand-sewn sutures. The incision line was then closed using a laparoscopic stapling device.

The tumors were removed in a bag (Endo Catch; Tyco Healthcare, Tokyo, Japan), and an air-leakage test was performed using endoscopic insufflation of the stomach. Anastomotic bleeding was evaluated using both endoscopy and laparoscopy and drainage tubes were inserted according to the situation.

7.4.5 Inverted LECS for GIST with Ulcerative Lesions (Figs. 7.7 and 7.9)

With the aim to appropriately resect the gastric wall, we developed LECS technique for the dissection of submucosal tumors of the stomach. Nunobe et al. used LECS in a case with laterally spreading intramucosal gastric cancer that fulfilled the extended criteria of ESD [13].

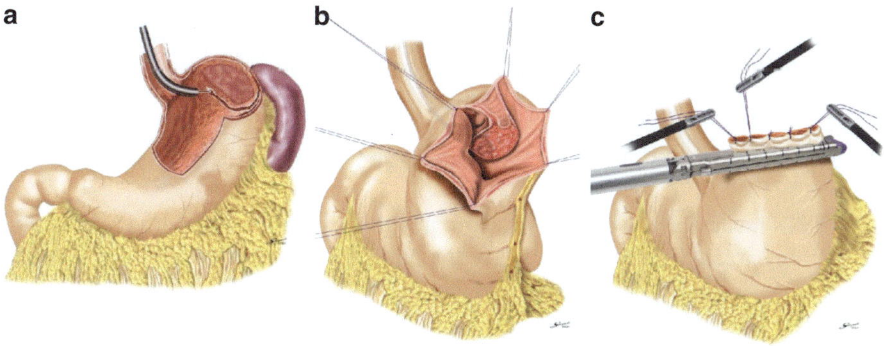

Fig. 7.7 Inverted LECS procedure (from reference [13] with permission). After circumferentially mucosal resection around the tumor (**a**), to prevent any contact with the visceral tissue, tumor is turned toward the intra-gastric cavity by pulling up of the resection line of the stomach like a bowel by several stiches (**b**). After the tumor has been resected, the edge of the incision line is temporarily closed using hand-sewn sutures. The incision line is then closed using a laparoscopic stapling device (**c**)

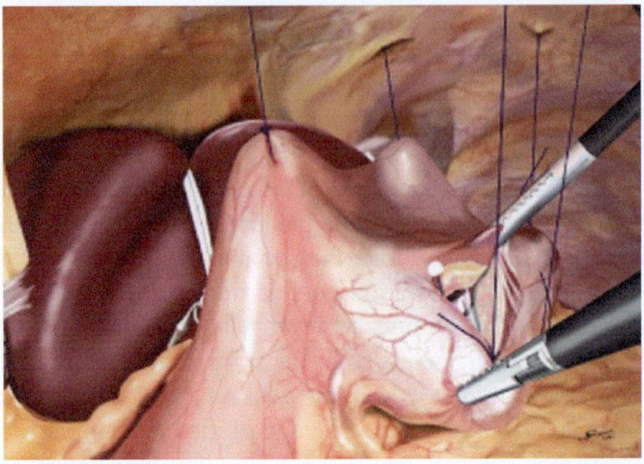

Fig. 7.8 Endoscopic dissection for the gastric wall during inverted LECS procedure (from reference [9] with permission). During the inverted LECS procedure, after circumferentially mucosal resection around the tumor, endoscopic operator mainly divide the seromuscular layer by the endoscopic device including IT-2 knife for preventing the tumor spilling over from the cavity of the stomach without tumor manipulation by the laparoscopic devices by the skillful endoscopic operator with sufficient ESD experiences

With LECS for epithelial neoplasms including GIST with ulcerative lesions, it is critical to ensure that no tumor cells are seeded in the peritoneal cavity. To prevent any contact with the visceral tissue, tumor is turned toward the intra-gastric cavity by pulling up of the resection line of the stomach like a bowel by several stiches. Recently, during the inverted LECS procedure, after circumferentially mucosal resection around the tumor, endoscopic operator mainly divide the seromuscular layer by the endoscopic device including IT-2 knife for preventing the tumor spilling over from the cavity of the stomach without tumor manipulation by the laparoscopic devices (Fig. 7.8). This technique is oncologically better procedure if possible by the skillful endoscopic operator with sufficient ESD experiences. Only gastric perforation during ESD for gastric cancer has been reported not to lead to peritoneal dissemination even with long-term observation [14] (Fig. 7.9).

7.4.6 LECS for GIST at the Esophagogastric Junction

For GISTs located at the esophagogastric junction, we believe that LECS is a good fit [12]. In cases where less than 1/3 of the circumference has been resected on the esophagogastric junction, it is believed that the cardia and its function can be spared (Fig. 7.10).

This shows the data on LECS used on the esophagogastric junction at our hospital (Table 7.1). It takes a little time to close after the resection, but it is believed that a better quality of life can be achieved after the procedure. If an invasion into the esophagus is discovered, the procedure is converted into a proximal gastrectomy as shown in the next section.

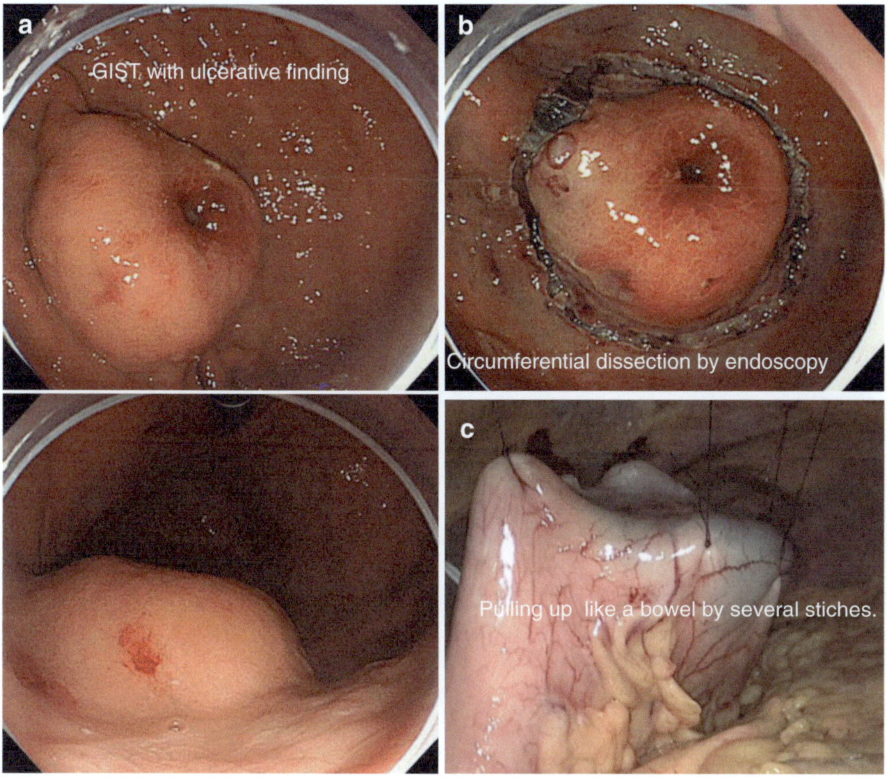

Fig. 7.9 Inverted LECS for the gastric GIST with ulcerative finding. After circumferential dissection by endoscopy for the gastric GIST with ulcerative finding (**a–c**), the gastric wall around the tumor is pulled up like a bowel by several stitches

For tumor located near the esophagogastric junction, closure of the gastric wall after tumor resection was performed using the laparoscopic hand-suturing technique more than a laparoscopic stapling device technique (Fig. 7.11). Recently, we have used the barbed suturing device for closing the gastric wall at the esophagogastric junction. It is essential point to reduce the reflux after surgery during the LECS for the esophagogastric tumor to make the His angle after anastomosis.

7.4.7 LECS Related Procedure [9]

To reduce the risk of cancer cell seeding through the open gastric wall, several full-thickness gastric wall resection approaches utilizing no exposure techniques such as the CLEAN-NET (Fig. 7.12) and the NEWS (Fig. 7.13) have been developed [15, 16].

Inoue et al. developed a method of non-exposed full-thickness resection after seromuscular incision, preserving the mucosa, which plays a role as a barrier. They refer to this technique as CLEAN-NET [15]. In this technique, after endoscopic

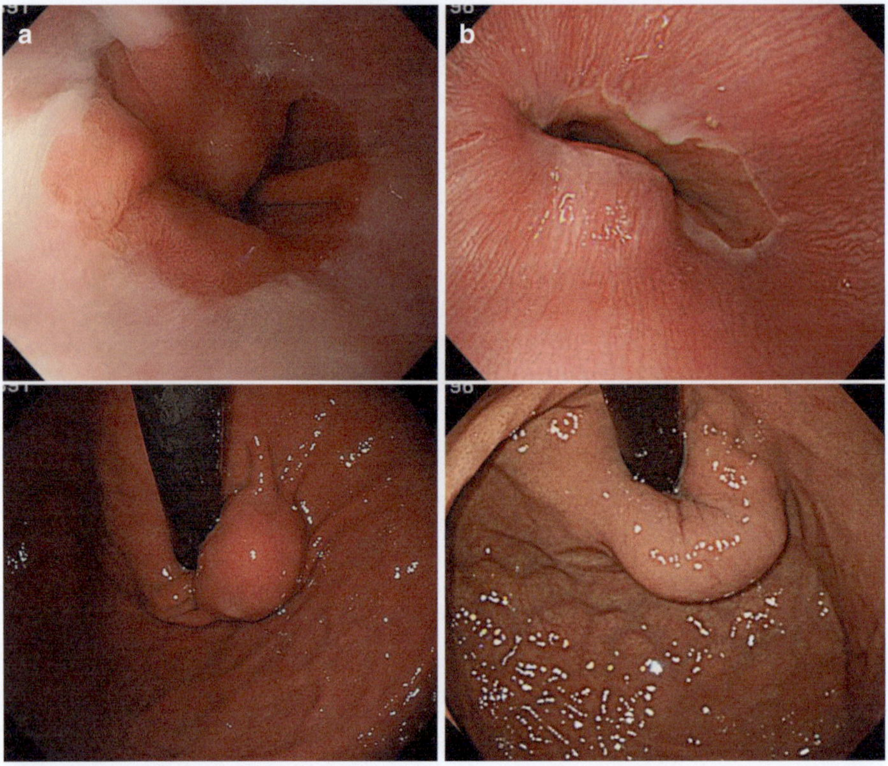

Fig. 7.10 Endoscopic findings for GIST at the esophagogastric junction: In cases where less than 1/3 of the circumference has been resected on the esophagogastric junction (**a**). In another case where more than 1/3 of the circumference, it is difficult to preserve the esophagogastric junction (**b**)

marking, four-layer stay sutures fix the mucosal layer to the seromuscular layer. The seromuscular layer is dissected laparoscopically along the outside of the stay sutures. The specimen is pulled up by stay sutures, and the mucosa surrounding the specimen is also lifted. The continuity of the mucosal layer prevents the gastric contents from flowing out into the peritoneal cavity. The full-layer specimen is resected with an adequate surgical margin using a laparoscopic stapling device. CLEAN-NET is a unique procedure and an attractive non-exposure technique for full-thickness resection of the gastric wall for gastric SMTs. However, if the tumor location is at the cardia, CLEAN-NET might be difficult to perform. Furthermore, in this procedure, the incision line is ultimately decided on from the serosal side, so, compared to classical LECS and inverted LECS procedure, determining the appropriate margin of the resection line might be difficult, because the gastric SMT including GIST is derived from muscular layer.

NEWS has been reported as a novel full-thickness resection technique without gastric perforation, aimed mainly at treating early gastric cancer [16]. In this procedure, mucosal marking is first placed around the tumor, followed by serosal marking via laparoscope under endoscopic navigation. Then, sodium hyaluronate solution

Table 7.1 LECS for the tumor at the esophagogastric junction in our hospital

	$N = 13$
Age (y. o.)	40.0 (18–72)
Sex (male: female)	6: 7
Size (mm)	32.0 (3–52)
Operation time (min)	293.0 (106–447)
Blood loss (ml)	10.7 (0–40)
Method of closure	
Stapler	4
Hand-sewn	9
Post-operative complication	
Stricture	0
Anastomotic failure	0
Reflux	0
Post-operative hospital stay (days)	9.0 (6–11)
Histopathological diagnosis	
GIST	5
Leiomyoma	7
NET (G1)	1
Surgical margin (positive: negative)	0: 13
Recurrence	none

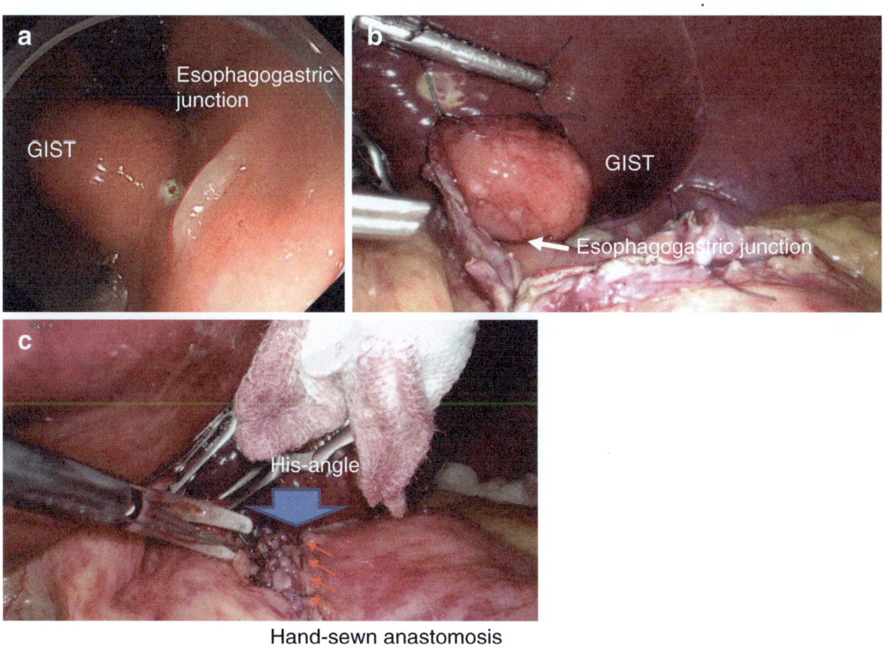

Fig. 7.11 LECS for the GIST at the esophagogastric junction: For tumor located near the esophagogastric junction (**a**, **b**), closure of the gastric wall after tumor resection is performed using the laparoscopic hand-suturing technique more than a laparoscopic stapling device technique (**c**). It is essential point to reduce the reflux after surgery during the LECS for the esophagogastric tumor to make the His angle after anastomosis

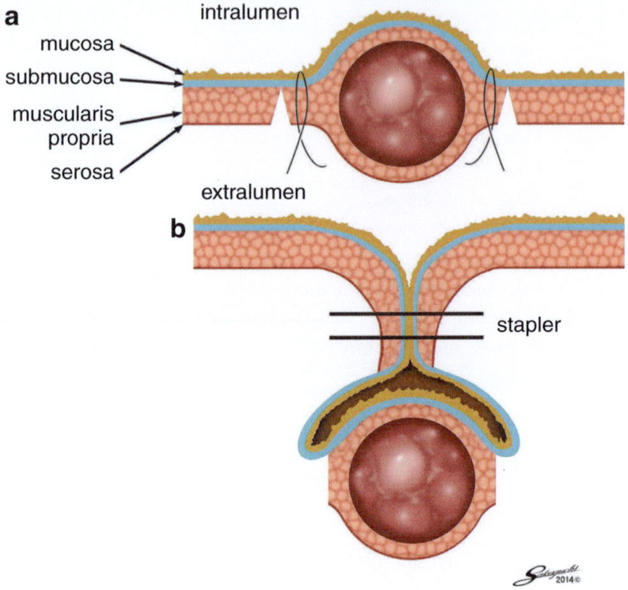

Fig. 7.12 CLEAN-NET as a LECS related procedure (from reference [9] with permission): Inoue et al. developed a method of non-exposed full-thickness resection after seromuscular incision, preserving the mucosa, which plays a role as a barrier. They refer to this technique as CLEAN-NET. In this technique, four-layer stay sutures fix the mucosal layer to the seromuscular layer. The seromuscular layer is dissected laparoscopically along the outside of the stay sutures (**a**). The specimen is pulled up by stay sutures, and the mucosa surrounding the specimen is also lifted. The continuity of the mucosal layer prevents the gastric contents from flowing out into the peritoneal cavity. The full-layer specimen is resected with an adequate surgical margin using a laparoscopic stapling device (**b**)

containing indigo carmine dye is injected into the submucosal layer circumferentially by endoscope. A circumferential seromuscular incision is performed laparoscopically around the serosal markings. The seromuscular layers are sutured, and the lesion is inverted into the inside of the stomach. During suturing, a laparoscopic surgical sponge is inserted to create a space between the suture layer and the serosal layer of the inverted lesion. This space provides a counter-traction to the mucosa and protects the suture line during the subsequent endoscopic resection. Finally, circumferential mucosal and submucosal tissue incisions are made endoscopically around the inverted tumor. The resected tumor and the spacer are retrieved perorally, and the mucosal defect is sutures with several endoscopic clips. As an advantage of this technique, both the serosal and mucosal layers can be resected precisely under direct visualization by laparoscopy or endoscopy. As to the indication of these non-exposure techniques, because the tumor would be orally collected via upper gastrointestinal tract, size of the tumor would be limited probably up to 3 cm in diameter. And, the location of the tumor would be also limited, for instance, at the esophagogastric junction.

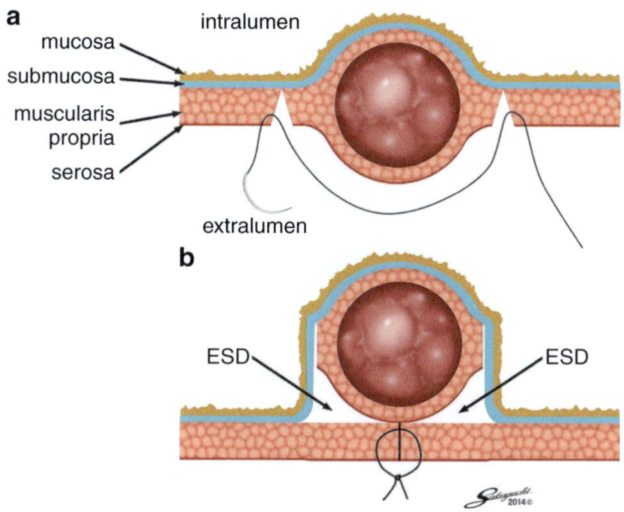

Fig. 7.13 NEWS as a LECS related procedure (from reference [9] with permission): NEWS has been reported as a novel full-thickness resection technique without gastric perforation, aimed mainly at treating early gastric cancer by Goto et al. In this procedure, mucosal marking is first placed around the tumor, followed by serosal marking via laparoscope under endoscopic navigation. Then, sodium hyaluronate solution containing indigo carmine dye is injected into the submucosal layer circumferentially by endoscope. A circumferential seromuscular incision is performed laparoscopically around the serosal markings (**a**). The seromuscular layers are sutured, and the lesion is inverted into the inside of the stomach (**b**). Finally, circumferential mucosal and submucosal tissue incisions are made endoscopically around the inverted tumor

7.5 Proximal Gastrectomy for GIST at the Esophagogastric Junction

LECS is a good fit for lesions located at the esophagogastric junction; however, a proximal gastrectomy is applied when the lesion covers more than 1/3 of the circumference on the esophagus side. At our hospital, we try the LECS procedure, and for cases where the resection is determined to be difficult during the procedure, we switch to a proximal gastrectomy. The removal of the lymph nodes is not normally necessary; therefore, the blood vessels along the gastric wall are manipulated and a proximal gastrectomy is completed. For large lesions in particular, grasping the tumor and working close to the cardia is assumed to be difficult, and the advantage of this procedure is thus to be able to resect the tumor as a package when it is a proximal gastrectomy.

The biggest problem with a proximal gastrectomy is reconstructive surgery.

Several reconstruction methods can be adopted after PG, including esophagogastrostomy, jejunal interposition (JI), and double-tract reconstruction. Esophagogastrostomy is the simplest reconstruction method; however, it is associated with a high risk of reflux esophagitis and gastroesophageal anastomotic stenosis. Tokunaga et al. conducted a questionnaire survey to evaluate these subjective

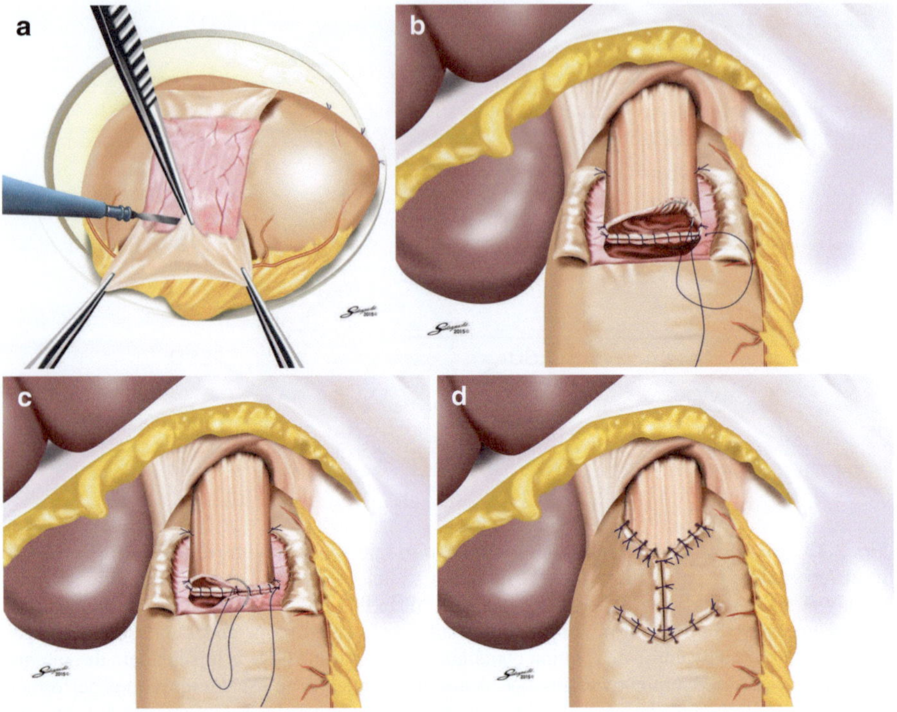

Fig. 7.14 Laparoscopic proximal gastrectomy with double-flap technique for the GIST at the esophagogastric junction (from reference [20] with permission): The remnant stomach was withdrawn from the umbilical incision and a 2.5 × 3.5 cm seromuscular double-flap was created on the anterior wall of the remnant stomach, leaving a region 1–2 cm from the proximal resection stump (**a**). Anastomosis is performed under laparoscopic guidance thereafter. First, the upper end of the flap is sutured to the posterior wall of the esophagus, usually with four stitches. The flap is then fixed 5 cm to the oral side of the portion of the esophagus intended for dissection while pulling up the esophagus stump. In doing so, the lower end of the esophagus is ultimately embedded within the stomach wall over a distance of 3–4 cm. Continuous sutures are applied through all layers of the posterior esophageal wall and the mucosa of the remnant stomach flap detachment surface (**b**). On the anterior wall, the esophagus and gastric wall at the lower end of the flap detachment surface is anastomosed layer-by-layer using interrupted sutures (**c**). To finish, the flap is positioned so that it covered the anastomosis site in a Y-shape, with the midline first anchored so that the flap covered the widest possible area (**d**)

symptoms after PG and determined that while JI might prevent endoscopic gastroesophageal reflux, it was also associated with higher incidence rates of subjective symptoms indicating delayed emptying [17]. Thus, the authors concluded that EG was a superior reconstruction method based on subjective symptoms and length of surgery. However, several issues remain to be resolved including endoscopic esophagitis during the post-operative period. In that regard, a promising reconstruction method after PG was laparoscopically performed recently in Japan; esophagogastrostomy was performed using a hand-sewn procedure, and the esophagogastric junction was reconstructed with the double-flap technique to prevent reflux (Figs. 7.14 and 7.15) [18–20]. The original procedure that formed the basis

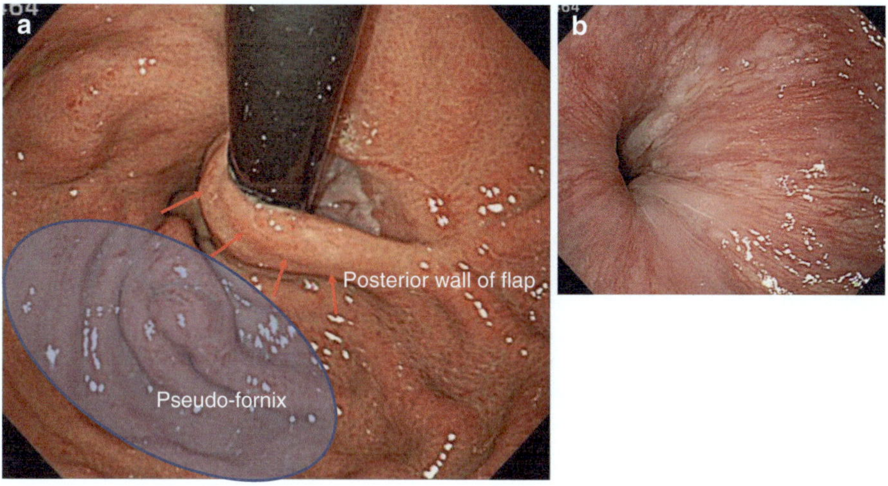

Fig. 7.15 Mechanism for prevention of reflux after laparoscopic proximal gastrectomy with double-flap technique: In this technique, the backflow valve is embedded between the submucosal layer and the seromuscular flap of the stomach, thus preventing backflow when compressed by resistance from intra-gastric pressure to the side and the flap from the anterior side (**a**). Endoscopic finding after laparoscopic proximal gastrectomy with double-flap shows no esophageal reflux (**b**)

for this method was designed for conventional open surgery. At our institute, we had favorable outcomes including morbidity and nutritional status after laparoscopic PG with the double-flap method compared with laparoscopic total gastrectomy [18].

7.6 Follow-Up After Surgery

The risk classification established in the NIH consensus conferences, the risk classification from the Armed Forces Institute of Pathology (AFIP) (Miettinen risk classification), and the modified Fletcher risk classification, such as Joensuu classification, are carefully reflected in the risk for reoccurrence. It is preferable that the follow-up after surgery is based on these risk classifications [1, 2]. For high risk or clinically malignant GIST cases, a CT scan follow-up is appropriate for the first 3 years once every 4–6 months, and then once a year until the 10th year after surgery. In GIST cases where there is a medium risk, low risk, or extremely low risk, we recommend a follow-up to be conducted every 6–12 months for the first 5 years after surgery and thereafter an abdominal CT scan once a year until the 10th year after surgery.

As a general rule, the post-operative follow-ups are based on the general principles for NIH risk classification. Yet, we believe that a detailed follow-up that is equal to or greater than a high risk classification is required for high risk GISTs with a high probability of reoccurrence, which refers to GISTs (clinically malignant GISTs) that are accompanied by even just one instance of a tumor rupture, hematogenous metastasis, disseminating lesion, or multiple organ invasion [21].

We believe that a CT scan is an appropriate means for a follow-up because reoccurrences after the resection are usually in the abdominal cavity; they are simple in nature; the inside of the abdominal cavity is spacious; the examination time is short; and the images are objective. The positive rate of GISTs in the PET-CT scan is not necessarily 100%, and the detection rate also of metastasis and dissemination is not necessarily higher than CT scans; therefore, we cannot say that the PET examination alone is useful.

References

1. Demetri GD, von Mehren M, Antonescu CR, et al. NCCN Task Force report: update on the management of patients with gastrointestinal stromal tumors. J Natl Compr Cancer Netw. 2010;8(Suppl 2):S1–S41.
2. The ESMO/European Sarcoma Network Working Group. Gastrointestinal stromal tumors: ESMO Clinical Practice Guidelines for diagnosis, treatment and follow-up. Ann Oncol. 2012;23(Supplement 7):vii49–55.
3. Fong Y, Coit DG, Woodruff JM, et al. Lymph node metastasis from soft tissue sarcoma in adults. Analysis of data from a prospective database of 1772 sarcoma patients. Ann Surg. 1993;217(1):72–7.
4. Eisenberg BL, Harris J, Blanke CD, et al. Phase II trial of neoadjuvant/adjuvant imatinib mesylate (IM) for advanced primary and metastatic/recurrent operable gastrointestinal stromal tumor (GIST): early results of RTOG 0132/ACRIN 6665. J Surg Oncol. 2009;99(1):42–7.
5. Wang D, Zhang Q, Blanke CD, et al. Phase II trial of neoadjuvant/adjuvant imatinib mesylate for advanced primary and metastatic/recurrent operable gastrointestinal stromal tumors: long-term follow-up results of Radiation Therapy Oncology Group 0132. Ann Surg Oncol. 2012;19(4):1074–780.
6. Hiki N, Yamamoto Y, Fukunaga T, Yamaguchi T, Nunobe S, Tokunaga M, Miki A, Ohyama S, Seto Y. Laparoscopic and endoscopic cooperative surgery for gastrointestinal stromal tumor dissection. Surg Endosc. 2008;22(7):1729–35.
7. Matsuda T, Hiki N, Nunobe S, et al. Feasibility of laparoscopic and endoscopic cooperative surgery for gastric submucosal tumors (with video). Gastrointest Endosc. 2015;84(1):47–52.
8. Matsuda T, Nunobe S, Kosuga T, Kawahira H, Inaki N, Kitashiro S, Abe N, Miyashiro I, Nagao S, Nishizaki M, Hiki N, Society for the study of Laparoscopy and Endoscopy Cooperative Surgery. Laparoscopic and luminal endoscopic cooperative surgery can be a standard treatment for submucosal tumors of the stomach: a retrospective multicenter study. Endoscopy. 2017;49(5):476–83.
9. Hiki N, Nunobe S, Matsuda T, et al. Laparoscopic endoscopic cooperative surgery. Dig Endosc. 2015;27(2):197–204.
10. Tsujimoto H, Yaguchi Y, Kumano I, et al. Successful gastric submucosal tumor resection using laparoscopic and endoscopic cooperative surgery. World J Surg. 2012;36(2):327–30.
11. Kawahira H, Hayashi H, Natsume T, et al. Surgical advantages of gastric SMTs by laparoscopy and endoscopy cooperative surgery. Hepato-Gastroenterology. 2012;59(114):415–7.
12. Hoteya S, Haruta S, Shinohara H, et al. Feasibility and safety of laparoscopic and endoscopic cooperative surgery for gastric submucosal tumors, including esophagogastric junction tumors. Dig Endosc. 2014;26(4):538–44.
13. Nunobe S, Hiki N, Gotoda T, et al. Successful application of laparoscopic and endoscopic cooperative surgery (LECS) for a lateral-spreading mucosal gastric cancer. Gastric Cancer. 2012;15(3):338–42.
14. Ikehara H, Gotoda T, Ono H, et al. Gastric perforation during endoscopic resection for gastric carcinoma and the risk of peritoneal dissemination. Br J Surg. 2007;94(8):992–5.

15. Inoue H, Ikeda H, Hosoya T, et al. Endoscopic mucosal resection, endoscopic submucosal dissection, and beyond: full-layer resection for gastric cancer with nonexposure technique (CLEAN-NET). Surg Oncol Clin N Am. 2012;21(1):129–40.
16. Goto O, Mitsui T, Fujishiro M, et al. New method of endoscopic full-thickness resection: a pilot study of non-exposed endoscopic wall-inversion surgery in an ex vivo porcine model. Gastric Cancer. 2011;14(2):183–7.
17. Tokunaga M, Hiki N, Ohyama S, et al. Effects of reconstruction methods on a patient's quality of life after a proximal gastrectomy: subjective symptoms evaluation using questionnaire survey. Langenbeck's Arch Surg. 2009;394:637–41.
18. Hayami M, Hiki N, Nunobe S, et al. Clinical outcomes and evaluation of laparoscopic proximal gastrectomy with double-flap technique for early gastric cancer in the upper third of the stomach. Ann Surg Oncol. 2017;24(6):1635–42.
19. Kuroda S, Nishizaki M, Kikuchi S, et al. Double-flap technique as an antireflux procedure in esophagogastrostomy after proximal gastrectomy. J Am Coll Surg. 2016;223(2):e7–e13.
20. Nunobe S, Hiki N. Function-preserving surgery for gastric cancer: current status and future perspectives. Transl Gastroenterol Hepatol. 2017;2:77. https://doi.org/10.21037/tgh.2017.09.07.
21. Takahashi T, Nakajima K, Nishitani A, et al. An enhanced risk-group stratification system for more practical prognostication of clinically malignant gastrointestinal stromal tumors. Int J Clin Oncol. 2007;12(5):369–74.

First-Line Treatment

8

Yusuke Onozawa

Abstract

Treatment of GIST has dramatically advanced due to the advent of imatinib. Treatment results improved with treatment using imatinib in advanced and recurrent GIST, with a handful of patients surviving without progression for longer than 10 years. The most important predictive factor of the effect of imatinib is a c-kit gene mutation, with a gene mutation of EXON11 being a good prognostic factor. In addition to this, the factor related to the effect of imatinib is the trough level of imatinib. Although the treatment results improved, primary resistant cases, in which the effect of imatinib cannot be expected from the beginning, and secondary resistant cases, in which the effect was exhibited at the beginning but resistance was exhibited later, have become problematic.

Keywords

Imatinib · c-Kit mutation

8.1 GIST Treatment Using Imatinib

No effective treatment for metastasis/recurrent GIST existed before 2000. Gain-of-function mutations of *c-kit* and *PDGFRA* genes were revealed to be involved in GIST development/proliferation mechanism. Imatinib was originally developed as a BCR-ABL inhibitor of chronic myelogenous leukemia (CML). At the molecular level, this drug binds to the ATP-binding part of BCR-ABL, KIT, and PDGFRA and inhibits all tyrosine kinase activities.

Y. Onozawa (✉)
Division of Medical Oncology, Shizuoka Cancer Center Hospital, Shizuoka, Japan
e-mail: y.onozawa@scchr.jp

Y. Kurokawa, Y. Komatsu (eds.), *Gastrointestinal Stromal Tumor*,
https://doi.org/10.1007/978-981-13-3206-7_8

After Joensuu from the University of Helsinki reported effective cases of imatinib against GIST in 2001, the development of treatment using imatinib rapidly advanced [1].

A phase I clinical trial of imatinib was conducted for patients with bone and soft tissue sarcomas including GIST by the EORTC Soft Tissue Sarcoma Group. It was administered in cohorts of 400 mg once daily, 300 mg twice daily, 400 mg twice daily, or 500 mg twice daily. As a result, 800 mg of imatinib per day was considered to be the maximum tolerated dose. Among these, objective effects were observed in 25 of 36 GIST patients (69%). Nineteen patients (53%) maintained PR and the rest maintained SD. Therapeutic effects were observed in all dose groups [2].

In the subsequent phase II clinical trial (B2222 study), 147 patients were treated at random in 400 mg/day or 600 mg/day imatinib treatment groups. Overall, 79 cases (53.7%) were radiographic response, 41 cases (27.9%) were stable disease, and seven cases (4.8%) could not be evaluated. Early resistance to imatinib was observed in 20 patients (13.6%). Treatment tolerability was good for both doses. No differences in toxicity or treatment effect were observed. At the initial reporting, the median follow-up period was 24 weeks and the median survival period was not reached. In a subsequent report, the median progression-free survival period was 24 months and the median overall survival period was 57 months [3]. An announcement of a follow-up period of 9 years was reported at ASCO in 2011. The median observation period was 9.4 years. Twenty-six patients (17.7%) continued treatment using imatinib. The overall survival rate over 9 years was 35%. Moreover, although it was long-term treatment for nearly 10 years, there were no serious adverse events reported in the follow-up until 3 years [4].

With the idea that more efficacy could be expected at higher doses, a random phase III trial using 400 mg versus 800 mg imatinib-administered groups was conducted among unresectable/metastatic GIST patients by a European group [5] and a US group. In the US trial, 694 people were randomized into two groups of 400 mg and 800 mg imatinib and compared. The median progression-free survival periods were 18 months in the 400 mg group and 20 months in the 800 mg group. The median overall survival periods were 55 months in the 400 mg group and 51 months in the 800 mg group [6]. At the ASCO announcement in 2014, 180 patients (26%) survived for more than 8 years and the 10-year survival rate was 22%. Approximately, half of the 137 long-term survivors continued treatment using imatinib.

This clinical trial failed to demonstrate a significant effect in the 800 mg group compared with the 400 mg group. Moreover, the toxicity was stronger in the 800 mg administration group. In this trial, in the event of disease progression in the 400 mg administration group, crossover to 800 mg administration was allowed. Among 118 patients for whom the treatment effect could be evaluated, partial remission was observed in three patients (3%) and stable disease was observed in 33 patients (28%). The median progression-free survival period after crossover was 3 months. Moreover, in the EXON 9 cases, the response rates were 17% in the 400 mg group and 67% in the 800 mg group, indicating a higher response rate in the 800 mg administration group. The median progression-free survival were also 9.4 months and 18.0 months, respectively, indicating significantly better results in the 800 mg administration group. However, no difference was observed in the median overall survival of 38.6 months and 38.4 months.

Crossover to 800 mg administration was also allowed in the phase III clinical trial conducted by the European group after exacerbation of the disease conditions in the 400 mg administration group. Among 133 patients who increased to 800 mg, partial remission was observed in three patients (3%), while no change was observed in 36 patients (27%), suggesting similar results. Although the usefulness of high-dose (800 mg/day) imatinib could not be demonstrated, it is important that clinical benefit can be obtained by increasing to 800 mg for 30% of patients whose disease conditions exacerbated at 400 mg/day [6].

An integrated analysis of these two trials was conducted. Overall, although the progression-free survival period was slightly longer in the 800 mg group, there was no difference in the overall survival period. Only in the EXON 9 mutation cases was the progression-free survival period of the 800 mg imatinib administration group prolonged (HR 0.58, 95% CI 0.38–0.91), in addition to having a significantly high response rate (47% versus 21%). In EXON 11 mutation cases, however, no differences were observed in either [7] (Table 8.1).

In the results of long-term follow-up recently reported in Europe, although it was an examination involving a small number of 62 cases, prolongation of the overall survival period was observed in EXON 9 mutation cases (HR 0.40, 95% CI 0.22–0.72) [8].

8.2 Impact of Pharmacokinetics on Imatinib Treatment

There are considerable individual differences in the pharmacokinetic exposure of imatinib which affect the clinical effect. Regarding the trough levels of imatinib in the plasma in a steady state in the study of the pharmacokinetics of imatinib in 73 patients with advanced and recurrent GIST, the minimum trough level was 414 ng/ml and the maximum trough level was 4182 ng/ml, revealing a significant difference of tenfold or more. The blood concentrations of these 73 patients were divided into four groups and the treatment effect was compared.

The clinical benefit rates indicating SD, PR, and CR were 12 of 18 patients (67%) in the Q1 group, which ranked in the bottom quartile, 29 of 36 patients (81%)

Table 8.1 Correlation of imatinib dose and tumor genotype with TTP and OS

		RR	TTP (months)	OS (months)
EXON 9	Imatinib 400 mg	17%	9.4	38.6
	Imatinib 800 mg	67%	18.0	38.4
EXON 11	Imatinib 400 mg	71%	27.2	60.0
	Imatinib 800 mg	72%	23.9	NR
WT	Imatinib 400 mg	42%	15.6	49.0
	Imatinib 800 mg	50%	9.8	39.5

TTP time to progression, *OS* overall survival, *IM 400* imatinib 400 mg daily, *IM800* imatinib 800 mg daily, *NR* not reached, *WT* wild type

Table 8.2 Correlation of imatinib plasma trough levels with response rate and time to progression

C min (ng/ml)	*n*	RR	TTP
<1110	18	44.8%	11.3 M
1110–2040	36	66.7%	30.6 M
2040<	19	73.3%	33.1 M

C min trough concentration, *RR* response rate, *TTP* time to progression

in the Q2 to Q3 groups, combining to make up the quartile below the median value (Q2 group) and quartile above the median value (Q3 group), and 16 of 19 patients (84%) in the Q4 group, which ranked in the top quartile. The clinical benefit rate in the Q2 to Q4 groups was 82%. Looking at the response rate which indicated an antitumor effect of PR or more, the response rates were 8 of 18 patients (44%) in the Q1 group, 24 of 36 patients (66.7%) in the Q2 to Q3 groups, and 14 of 19 (73.3%) in the Q4 group. While the progression-free period was 11.3 months in the Q1 group, it was 30.6 months in the Q2 to Q3 groups, and 33.1 months in the Q4 group. No significant differences were observed in the overall survival.

In the Q1 group whose blood concentration was in the bottom quartile (trough level was less than 1110 ng/ml), the clinical effect rate was low and the disease progression-free survival time was short. The trough level in a steady state is important in terms of the antitumor effect of imatinib [9] (Table 8.2).

In the study of blood concentrations of 92 patients taking 400 mg/day of imatinib, the histories of major gastrectomy, serum Alb, and creatinine clearance were factors impacting the trough level of imatinib [10].

8.3 Effect of Gene Mutations on Imatinib Treatment

It is most important to evaluate gene mutations when predicting the treatment effect and prognosis of imatinib. The responses to imatinib treatment vary depending on the genotype of GIST.

c-Kit and PDGFRA mutations observed in many GIST patients are related to the treatment effect of imatinib.

The c-kit gene mutation is related to the treatment effect and prognosis of imatinib. Heinrich et al. reported on 127 cases in which KIT and PDGFRA mutations were examined in the B2222 study. The response rate of imatinib was high in GIST patients with the EXON 11 mutation compared to patients with the EXON 9 mutation and patients without mutations in kit (83.5% vs 47.8% vs 0%) along with significantly long event-free survival [11].

Moreover, Heinrich et al. also conducted similar studies in another clinical trial, comparing GIST patients with the EXON 11 mutation to patients with the EXON 9 mutation and wild-type patients. The response rates were 71.7% vs 44.4% vs 44.6%, the progression-free survival periods were 24.7 months vs 16.7 months vs 12.8 months, and the median overall survival periods were 60 months vs 38.4 months vs 49.0 months. The treatment effect of imatinib and prognosis were good in GIST

Table 8.3 Clinical benefit rate for patients with KIT EXON 11 and EXON 9 mutations by imatinib plasma trough levels

C min (ng/ ml)	EXON 9/11	RR	CR + PR + SD
<1110	3/9	0%/67%	67%/67%
1110–2040	8/17	50%/84%	62.5%/100%
2040<	1/13	0%/92%	100%/100%

CR complete response, *PR* partial response, *SD* stable disease, C_{min} trough concentration

patients with EXON 11 mutations, giving consistent results with the other study [7, 9] (Table 8.3).

GIST indicating primary resistance, in which the disease conditions become worse within 6 months after imatinib treatment, makes up approximately 10–15% of the total. Most of these cases do not have KIT and PDGFRA genetic mutations, have the PDGFRA gene D842V mutation, or are succinate dehydrogenase (SDH)-deficient GISTs. Imatinib treatment should not be conducted for these GISTs. Many of these GISTs are KIT negative upon immunostaining. However, among KIT-negative GISTs upon immunostaining, PDGFRA mutant GISTs other than D842V are also included, and therefore KIT negative upon immunostaining does not rule out imatinib treatment.

Neurofibromatosis type 1 (NF1), which is a disease caused by NF1 gene mutation, increases the risk of GIST. In GISTs of these patients, although KIT is expressed upon immunostaining, KIT or PDGFRA genes mutation is not observed. Moreover, imatinib has little effect on these GISTs.

The treatment results of imatinib for 31 patients with PDGFRA D842V mutation GIST demonstrated no responder and 21 disease progression (68%) in terms of the best treatment effect [12]. Although this was a limited report, the response cases of regorafenib and dasatinib were reported [13].

There was one PR case in the imatinib treatment for 49 patients with succinate dehydrogenase (SDH)-deficient GIST. However, the progress of the succinate dehydrogenase-deficient GIST was slow. In the study of 63 patients with succinate dehydrogenase-deficient GIST, only three patients were found to have died due to exacerbation of disease conditions at the median observation period of 6 years [14].

Regarding these GISTs, no optimal treatment has been established. They may be good candidates for clinical trials including phase I clinical trials.

8.4 Conclusion

Most cases of GISTs have a kit gene mutation and are involved in tumor cell proliferation. With the appearance of imatinib, which inhibits the phosphorylation of c-kit, the treatment of GIST has dramatically changed. Treatment with 400 mg oral imatinib is the standard treatment in the first treatment of unresectable/recurrent GIST as of now.

The c-kit gene mutation is the predictive factor regarding the effect of imatinib. GIST with the EXON 9 mutation indicates a poor prognosis compared to GIST with the EXON 11 mutation; however, improvements in the progression-free survival period and response rate are demonstrated with an oral dose of 800 mg.

In addition, the blood concentration trough level of imatinib affects the effect of imatinib.

In the event of early worsening with imatinib treatment, it is necessary to consider GISTs having a genetic mutation on which imatinib has no effect.

References

1. Joensuu H, Roberts P, Sarlomo-Rikkala M, Andersson LC, Tervaharatiala P, Silberman S, Capdeville R, Dimitrlievic S, Druker B, Demetri GD. Safety and efficacy of imatinib (STI571) in metastatic gastrointestinal stromal tumors. N Engl J Med. 2001;344(14):1052–6.
2. van Oosterom AT, Judson I, Verweij J, Stroobants S, di Paola ED, Dimitrijevic S, Martens M, Webb A, Sciot R, Van Glabbeke M, Silberman S, Nielsen OS. Safety and efficacy of imatinib (STI571) in metastatic gastrointestinal stromal tumours: a phase I study. Lancet. 2001;358(9291):1421–3.
3. Demetri GD, von Mehren M, Blanke CD, Van den Abbeele AD, Eisenberg B, Roberts PJ, Heinrich MC, et al. Efficacy and safety of imatinib (STI571) in advanced gastrointestinal stromal tumors. N Engl J Med. 2002;347(7):472.
4. Patel S. Long-term efficacy of imatinib for treatment of metastatic GIST. Cancer Chemother Pharmacol. 2013;72(2):277–86.
5. Verweij J, Casali PG, Zalcberg J, LeCesne A, Reichardt P, Blay J-Y, Issels R, van Oosterom A, Hogendoorn PCW, Van Glabbeke M, Bertulli R, Judson I. Progression-free survival in gastrointestinal stromal tumours with high-dose imatinib: randomised trial. Lancet. 2004;364(9440):1127–34.
6. Blanke CD, Rankin C, Demetri GD, Ryan CW, von Mehren M, Benjamin RS, Raymond AK, Bramwell VH, Baker LH, Maki RG, Tanaka M, Hecht JR, Heinrich MC, Fletcher CD, Crowley JJ, Borden EC. Phase III randomized, intergroup trial assessing imatinib mesylate at two dose levels in patients with unresectable or metastatic gastrointestinal stromal tumors expressing the kit receptor tyrosine kinase: S0033. J Clin Oncol. 2008;26(4):626–32.
7. Heinrich MC, Owzar K, Corless CL, Hollis D, Borden EC, Fletcher CD, Ryan CW, von Mehren M, Blanke CD, Rankin C, Benjamin RS, Bramwell VH, Demetri GD, Bertagnolli MM, Fletcher JA. Correlation of kinase genotype and clinical outcome in the North American Intergroup Phase III Trial of imatinib mesylate for treatment of advanced gastrointestinal stromal tumor: CALGB 150105 Study by Cancer and Leukemia Group B and Southwest Oncology Group. J Clin Oncol. 2008;26(33):5360–7.
8. Casali PG, Zalcberg J, Le Cesne A, Reichardt P, Blay JY, Lindner LH, Judson IR, Schoffski P, Leyvraz S, Italiano A, Grunwald V, Pousa AL, Kotasek D, Sleijfer S, Kerst JM, Rutkowski P, Fumagalli E, Hogendoorn P, Litiere S, Marreaud S, van der Graaf W, Gronchi A, Verweij J, European Organisation for, R, Treatment of Cancer Soft, T, Bone Sarcoma Group, I S G, Australasian Gastrointestinal Trials, G. Ten-year progression-free and overall survival in patients with unresectable or metastatic GI stromal tumors: long-term analysis of the European Organisation for Research and Treatment of Cancer, Italian Sarcoma Group, and Australasian Gastrointestinal Trials Group Intergroup Phase III Randomized Trial on Imatinib at Two Dose Levels. J Clin Oncol. 2017;35(15):1713–20.
9. Demetri GD, Wang Y, Wehrle E, Racine A, Nikolova Z, Blanke CD, Joensuu H, von Mehren M. Imatinib plasma levels are correlated with clinical benefit in patients with unresectable/metastatic gastrointestinal stromal tumors. J Clin Oncol. 2009;27(19):3141–7.

10. Yoo C, Ryu MH, Kang BW, Yoon SK, Ryoo BY, Chang HM, Lee JL, Beck MY, Kim TW, Kang YK. Cross-sectional study of imatinib plasma trough levels in patients with advanced gastrointestinal stromal tumors: impact of gastrointestinal resection on exposure to imatinib. J Clin Oncol. 2010;28(9):1554–9.
11. Heinrich MC, Corless CL, Demetri GD, Blanke CD, von Mehren M, Joensuu H, McGreevey LS, Chen CJ, Van den Abbeele AD, Druker BJ, Kiese B, Eisenberg B, Roberts PJ, Singer S, Fletcher CD, Silberman S, Dimitrijevic S, Fletcher JA. Kinase mutations and imatinib response in patients with metastatic gastrointestinal stromal tumor. J Clin Oncol. 2003;21(23):4342–9.
12. Cassier PA, Fumagalli E, Rutkowski P, Schoffski P, Van Glabbeke M, Debiec-Rychter M, Emile JF, Duffaud F, Martin-Broto J, Landi B, Adenis A, Bertucci F, Bompas E, Bouche O, Leyvraz S, Judson I, Verweij J, Casali P, Blay JY, Hohenberger P, European Organisation for, R, Treatment of, C. Outcome of patients with platelet-derived growth factor receptor alpha-mutated gastrointestinal stromal tumors in the tyrosine kinase inhibitor era. Clin Cancer Res. 2012;18(16):4458–64.
13. Kollàr A, Maruzzo M, Messiou C, Cartwright E, Miah A, Martin-Liberal J, Thway K, McGrath E, Dunlop A, Khabra K, Seddon B, Dileo P, Linch M, Judson I, Benson C. Regorafenib treatment for advanced, refractory gastrointestinal stromal tumor: a report of the UK managed access program. Clin Sarcoma Res. 2014;17(4):17.
14. Boikos SA, Pappo AS, Killian JK, LaQuaglia MP, Weldon CB, George S, Trent JC, von Mehren M, Wright JA, Schiffman JD, Raygada M, Pacak K, Meltzer PS, Miettinen MM, Stratakis C, Janeway KA, Helman LJ. Molecular subtypes of KIT/PDGFRA wild-type gastrointestinal stromal tumors: a report from the National Institutes of Health Gastrointestinal Stromal Tumor Clinic. JAMA Oncol. 2016;2(7):922–8.

Second- and Third-Line Treatment

9

Masato Ozaka

Abstract

Sunitinib (sunitinib malate; SU11248) is a novel oral multitargeted tyrosine kinase inhibitor with antitumor and antiangiogenic activities. Sunitinib has been identified as a potent inhibitor of VEGFR-1, VEGFR-2, fetal liver tyrosine kinase receptor 3 (FLT3), KIT (stem-cell factor [SCF] receptor), PDGFRα, and PDGFR. Regorafenib is a small molecule inhibitor of multiple membrane-bound and intracellular kinases involved in normal cellular functions and in pathologic processes such as oncogenesis, tumor angiogenesis, and maintenance of the tumor microenvironment. Regorafenib blocks the activity of several protein kinases involved with angiogenesis (vascular endothelial growth factor [VEGF] receptors 1–3 and TIE2), oncogenesis (KIT, RET, RAF1, B-RAF, and B-RAF V600E), and the tumor microenvironment (platelet-derived growth factor receptor [PDGFR] and fibroblast growth factor receptors [FGFR]). Sunitinib and Regorafenib are two targeted agents with worldwide approval for second- and third-line treatment, respectively, in metastatic GIST.

Keywords

GIST · Sunitinib · Regorafenib · Imatinib resistance

M. Ozaka (✉)
Department of Gastroenterology, The Cancer Institute Hospital of JFCR, Tokyo, Japan
e-mail: masato.ozaka@jfcr.or.jp

Y. Kurokawa, Y. Komatsu (eds.), *Gastrointestinal Stromal Tumor*,
https://doi.org/10.1007/978-981-13-3206-7_9

9.1 Second-Line Treatment

9.1.1 Sunitinib

9.1.1.1 Mechanism of Action

Sunitinib (sunitinib malate; SU11248) is a novel oral multitargeted tyrosine kinase inhibitor with antitumor and antiangiogenic activities. Sunitinib has been identified as a potent inhibitor of VEGFR-1, VEGFR-2, fetal liver tyrosine kinase receptor 3 (FLT3), KIT (stem-cell factor [SCF] receptor), PDGFRα, and PDGFRβ in both biochemical and cellular assays [1]. In vitro, sunitinib inhibited the growth of cell lines driven by VEGF, SCF, and PDGF and induced apoptosis of human umbilical vein endothelial cells. In vivo, sunitinib caused bone marrow depletion and effects in the pancreas in rats and monkeys, as well as adrenal toxicity in rat (micro hemorrhage) [2]. In monkeys, a slight increase in arterial blood pressure and QT interval was reported at higher doses. Sunitinib exhibited dose- and time-dependent antitumor activity in mice, potently repressing the growth of a broad variety of human tumor xenografts.

9.1.1.2 Pharmacological Parameters

Sunitinib is metabolized primarily by the cytochrome P450 enzyme, CYP3A4, to produce its primary active metabolite [*N*-desethyl metabolite (SU012662)]. SU012662 is considered equipotent to the parent compound regarding the inhibition of VEGFR, PDGFR, and KIT [2–5]. In a human mass balance study of sunitinib, 61% of the dose was eliminated in feces, with renal elimination accounting for 16% of the administered dose. Sunitinib and its primary active metabolite were the major drug-related compounds identified in plasma, urine, and feces, representing 91.5%, 86.4%, and 73.8% of radioactivity in pooled samples, respectively. Minor metabolites were identified in urine and feces but generally not found in plasma. Total oral clearance ranged from 34 to 62 L/h with an inter-patient variability of 40%.

9.1.1.3 Clinical Trial

Preclinical

Molecular mechanisms by sunitinib that exerts its antitumor function are not clearly elucidated, partly because available preclinical data are scarce. Preclinical studies with GIST cell lines suggest that SU11248 induces growth arrest and apoptosis of GIST cells. In addition, GIST cells exposition to SU11248 inhibits c-KIT autophosphorylation and the phosphorylation of AKT and ERK, key components of PI3K-Akt-mTOR and MAPK pathways, respectively, involved in cell survival and proliferation. This fact provides a rational for combining sunitinib with other target therapies directed to the mentioned pathways [6].

Phase I/II

An open-label, single-arm, dose escalation phase I/II trial in Western population enrolled 97 patients with metastatic GIST who have progressed to imatinib or they were intolerant to it [7]. Several doses and schedules were tested in different cohorts in order to evaluate treatment safety: schedule 2/2 (2 weeks ON sunitinib, 2 weeks OFF) at doses of 25, 50, or 75 mg/day, and schedules 4/2 and 2/1 starting at 50 mg/day. The dose of 50 mg/day was defined as maximum tolerated dose because two of four patients treated at 75 mg/day 2/2 experienced dose-limiting toxicities during the first cycle (fatigue, nausea, and vomiting). Pharmacokinetic analysis revealed that steady-state was achieved by days 7–10 and 7–21 for sunitinib and SU12662, respectively. In order to maximize sunitinib exposure, the schedule 4/2 was selected for further development. Promising sunitinib activity was observed in this trial since 54% of patients benefited from the treatment. More concisely, 7 patients presented PR with a median time of 8.3 months to achieve it and 45 patients experienced long-lasting stable disease for a minimum of 6 months. Median PFS was 7.8 months (95% condense interval [CI], 5.1–10.4 months), and median OS was 19 months (95% CI, 12.9–21.5 months). Approximately 60 participants of this trial had a baseline positron emission tomography with 18Fluorodeoxyglucose (FDG-PET) and another on day 7 of cycle 1. Even if it will be detailed later, early metabolic responses correlated with better clinical outcomes.

In addition, sunitinib activity was also demonstrated in a preclinical setting because approximately half of the patients included had pre- and post-sunitinib biopsies. After 1 week of sunitinib treatment, levels of phospho-KIT in tumor samples as well as the expression of proteins involved in cell proliferation (cyclin A and AKT) in a percentage of patients were reduced. Mentioned early changes related to lower cell proliferation could correlate with better clinical outcomes, but it is a hypothesis to be further demonstrated.

Another phase I/II nonrandomized, open-label, and dose-escalating study aimed to evaluate the safety and preliminary efficacy of sunitinib in Asiatic population [8]. About 12 patients were enrolled in part I and doses of 25, 50, and 75 mg/day of sunitinib on schedule 4/2 were tested; 50 mg/day on schedule 4/2 until progression disease and/or unacceptable toxicity was designed as recommended phase II dose and after that several dose-limiting toxicities were observed in the cohort of 75 mg/day on schedule 4/2. A total of 36 patients were included in part II of the study and received the previously defined dose. According to response evaluation criteria in solid tumors (RECIST), 11% of patients experiment a PR and the disease control rate was ~61%. Median TTP was 28.3 weeks. Regarding safety, all patients included experienced at least one adverse treatment-related event, but 84% of them were grade 1/2 and generally manageable and reversible (Table 9.1).

Table 9.1 Efficacy of sunitinib and regorafenib in trials with patients treated for GIST

	Sunitinib		Regorafenib
	Phase I [8]	Phase III [9]	Phase III [10]
	$n = 97$	$n = 207$	$n = 133$
ORR	8(8%)	17(8%)	6(4.5%)
SD	36(37%)	37(18%)	95(71.4%)
TTP/PFS	7.8M	6.3M	4.8M
OS	19.8M	NR	NR

Phase III

After phase I/II trial, sunitinib efficacy was further demonstrated in a phase III trial [11]. This one was multicenter, randomized, double-blind, and placebo-controlled in patients who had presented imatinib resistance or intolerance. A total of 302 patients were randomly assigned 2:1 to receive sunitinib at doses established in phase I (*n*: 207) or placebo (*n*: 105). However, the trial was early unblinded due to the results of planned interim analysis that clearly favored sunitinib in terms of TTP. Median TTP in sunitinib arm was 27.3 weeks (95% CI 16.0–32.1) versus 6.4 weeks in placebo ones (95% CI 4.4–10.0; hazard ratio [HR] 0.33; 95% CI 0.23–0.47; $P = 0.001$). After these results, all patients treated with placebo were allowed to receive open-label sunitinib. OS data were more difficult to analyze because of the crossover. According to Kaplan–Meier method, OS did not reveal statistically significant differences between sunitinib and placebo (73.9 weeks versus 64.9 weeks; 95% CI 45.7–96.0; $P = 0.161$). Nonetheless, a posterior long-term OS analysis was performed using another statistical method that accounts for the bias introduced by the crossover from placebo to sunitinib, the rank-preserving structural failure time (RPSFT). RPSFT method identified clear differences in median OS favoring sunitinib group (73.9 weeks; 95% CI 61.3–85.7 versus 35.7 weeks; 95% CI 25.7–49.8; $P = 0.001$) [9, 12].

9.1.1.4 Safety

In a phase I/II trial with sunitinib in patients with imatinib-resistant/-intolerant GIST (*N* 97), the most commonly reported treatment-related AEs were grade 1–2 fatigue, diarrhea, skin discoloration, nausea, and hand–foot syndrome. Treatment-related grade 3–4 AEs included hypertension (17%), asymptomatic lipase increase (13%), and fatigue (10%). Eight patients (8%) discontinued treatment due to AEs.

In a phase III randomized controlled trial of sunitinib in patients (*N* 312) with imatinib-resistant/-intolerant advanced GIST, treatment-related AEs were reported in 83% (*n* 168) of patients in the sunitinib group and 59% (*n* 60) in the placebo group [9, 11]. An updated analysis of this study (*N* 361; *n* 243, sunitinib; *n* 118, placebo) reported the incidence of treatment-related AEs for the blinded, unblinded, and overall populations [13]. The profile of AE observed was similar to that of the phase I/II study. Moreover, similar incidences of AEs were observed in the blinded and unblinded populations. A slightly higher incidence of non-hematological AEs was noted with longer duration of sunitinib therapy. Treatment-related hypothyroidism (all grades) was reported in 13% of patients. Most hematological laboratory abnormalities were grade 1–2 and were similar in frequency to those occurring with shorter-term sunitinib therapy (Table 9.2).

9.1.1.5 Alternative Schedules of Sunitinib

Alternative schemes of sunitinib have been investigated in order to improve the safety profile and tolerance [14]. Sunitinib 37.5 mg once daily until PD and/or unacceptable toxicity were evaluated in an open-label, multicenter, phase II trial in which patients were randomized in a ratio of 1:1 in order to receive the mentioned

Table 9.2 Grade 3 or 4 toxicity of sunitinib and regorafenib in trials with patients treated for GIST

	Sunitinib		Regorafenib
	$n = 97$	$n = 207$	$n = 133$
Fatigue	10%	7%	1.50%
Diarrhea	7%	4%	5.30%
Nausea	4%	1%	0.80%
Dermatitis	7%	5%	19.70%
Stomatitis	3%	NA	1.50%
Lipase increase	13%	NA	NA
Hypertension	17%	4%	22.70%
Neutropenia	NA	8%	NA
Anemia	NA	4%	NA
Thrombocytopenia	NA	5%	30%

dose in the morning or in the evening [13]. The results of this trial in terms of both efficacy and toxicity overlapped with the phase III patients, with a median PFS of 34 weeks (95% CI, 24–49) and a median OS of 107 weeks (95% CI, 72 to not calculable). Consequently, sunitinib 37.5 mg once daily could be considered as an alternative dosing strategy, although it has not been directly compared with standard scheme. Regarding the optimal condition in sunitinib intake, no major differences were found between morning and evening dosing. In both the cases, no drug accumulation was observed across cycles and effective drug concentration was achieved.

Sunitinib 50 mg/daily in a schedule of 2 weeks ON/1 week OFF has been investigated in metastatic renal cell carcinoma. The RESTORE trial accrued 76 patients, and they were randomized to sunitinib 4 weeks ON/2 weeks OFF schedule or to the 2 weeks ON/1-week OFF regimen [15]. The results of this trial demonstrated better toxicity profile and better compliance with the 2/1 schedule. A retrospective analysis with 249 patients concluded with similar results [16]. Even though this scheme has not been evaluated in GIST patients, it could be considered in some patients with poor tolerance to the conventional schedule [17].

9.1.1.6 Surgery After Sunitinib Treatment

Unless treatment with sunitinib in metastatic GIST patients should be considered as palliative, a potentially radical surgery could be occasionally planned in the clinical practice if the response has been good enough. Nonetheless, the scientific evidence supporting this surgical management is very scarce. Two retrospective series with a very limited number of patients (10 and 50) suggest that post-sunitinib surgery is feasible, but the patients should be selected carefully because no clear improvement in terms of survival has been suggested. In addition, in the largest series, the surgery was frequently incomplete (not clearly related with the magnitude of the previous sunitinib response) and significant complications occurred in >50% of patients [18–20].

9.1.1.7 Mutational Status

Refractory GIST is a heterogeneous disease composed of a mixture of clones; each of them harbors different mutations mainly in KIT or PDGFRA. Despite every lesion in a given patient has the primary GIST mutation (except of wild-type GIST), secondary mutations can appear under treatment pressure and confer resistance to therapies. The percentage of secondary mutations in GIST with primary mutations is estimated to range between 44% and 90%, depending on the sensitivity of the method used to determine them. In addition, the development of several secondary mutations at the same time seems to be a common event. After imatinib exposure, secondary mutations are more commonly found in GIST with primary KIT exon 11 mutations than in GIST with primary KIT exon 9 mutations and not found in GIST wild-type. Secondary mutations after imatinib treatment are usually located at exons 13 (for example, V654A mutation) and 14 (for example, T607I mutation), both encode the ATP-binding pocket, or in exon 17 (encodes kinase activation loop) [21].

The potential role of primary and secondary mutations as predictor factors of sunitinib response has been investigated. A retrospective analysis using samples from patients who are included in a phase I/II sunitinib trial concluded that patients with KIT exon 9 mutations clearly benefited more of sunitinib than those patients who harbor KIT exon 11 mutations in terms of objective response rate (37% versus 5%; $P = 0.002$), PFS (19.4 months versus 5.1 months; $P = 0.0005$), and OS (26.9 months versus 12.3 months; $P = 0.012$). These results have also been reported in a series of 137 patients in whose tumors carried KIT exon 9 mutations or were wild-type and presented clearly better 1-year PFS compared with those whose tumors carried a KIT exon 11 or PDGFRA mutations (68% and 57% versus 34% and 15%, respectively). $KIT^{AY502\text{-}3ins}$ mutations at exon 9 is the most sensitive to sunitinib [22].

Regarding secondary mutations, in vitro studies with GIST cell lines suggest that sunitinib is highly active against kinase activity of KIT containing secondary mutations at ATP-binding pocket (exons 13 and 14), in contrast to GIST cell lines harboring imatinib resistant mutations at activation loop (exon 17, for example, D820Y, D820E, and NK822K, and exon 18). These findings correlate with better PFS and OS of patients treated with sunitinib with exon 13 and 14 mutations, compared with patients with exon 17 and 18 mutations, although these results should be further validated.

The 10–15% of GIST patients defined as "wild-type" (WT, no mutations in KIT neither in PDGFRA) are of special interest, since the vast majority do not respond to imatinib. In these cases, the deficiency of succinate dehydrogenase (due to either inactivating mutations or through epigenetic mechanisms) [23] and sporadic mutations in the MAPK pathway have a major role in tumor development. Among pediatric population, GIST WT is the most frequently found, sporadically or as a part of congenital syndromes such as Carney triad or neurofibromatosis type 1. In this subset of patients, sunitinib shows promising substantial antitumor activity and acceptable tolerability. In addition, preclinical data suggest higher antitumor efficacy of sunitinib compared with imatinib [23, 24].

9.2 Third-Line Treatment

9.2.1 Regorafenib

9.2.1.1 Mechanism of Action

Regorafenib is a small molecule inhibitor of multiple membrane-bound and intracellular kinases involved in normal cellular functions and in pathologic processes such as oncogenesis, tumor angiogenesis, and maintenance of the tumor microenvironment. Regorafenib blocks the activity of several protein kinases involved with angiogenesis (vascular endothelial growth factor [VEGF] receptors 1–3 and TIE2), oncogenesis (KIT, RET, RAF1, B-RAF, and B-RAF V600E), and the tumor microenvironment (platelet-derived growth factor receptor [PDGFR] and fibroblast growth factor receptors [FGFR]) [25, 26].

9.2.1.2 Pharmacological Parameters

Regorafenib is metabolized by CYP3A4 and UGT1A9. The main circulating metabolites of regorafenib measured at steady-state in human plasma are M-2 (*N*-oxide) and M-5 (*N*-oxide and *N*-desmethyl), both of them having similar in vitro pharmacological activity and steady-state concentrations as regorafenib. M-2 and M-5 are highly protein bound (99.8% and 99.95%, respectively).

9.2.1.3 Clinical Trial

Phase I

Several phase I studies have been performed with regorafenib. Mross and colleagues enrolled 53 subjects (16 with colorectal cancer) in an open-label, nonrandomized, dose-escalating phase I study using oral doses of 10–220 mg daily. The dose-limiting toxicities were found to be hand–foot skin reaction, rash, abdominal pain, and asthma seen at the dose of 220 mg dose level.

Another phase I dose escalation trial enrolled 38 subjects with advanced solid tumors (colorectal 16%) and used doses of 20–140 mg. The maximum tolerated dose in this study was 100 mg orally daily every 21 days, continuously.

Strumberg and colleagues also studied 38 subjects with refractory mCRC in a phase I dose escalation study. Patients enrolled on the dose escalation portion trial received doses of 60–220 mg/day of regorafenib. Based on the positive results of the dose escalation portion of this trial, additional mCRC patients were enrolled in an extension of the trial. These patients received 160 mg orally daily for 21 out of 28 days. The most common toxicities seen were hand–foot skin reactions, fatigue, voice change, and rash. A total of 27 patients were evaluable for response; of these 74% showed some disease control with regorafenib treatment.

Awada and colleagues investigated a different schedule of administration of regorafenib in their phase I trial. Patients received treatment in a 28-day cycle with 21 days of regorafenib treatment followed by 7 days off. Patients received oral doses of 10–120 mg daily. Pharmacokinetic and pharmacodynamic parameters as well as tumor response were evaluated in 44 patients with solid tumors. PK parameters showed a linear association with dose and PD parameters correlated with dose exposure. Partial response and stable disease were achieved in two and four patients, respectively. The dose-limiting toxicity was reported in patients receiving the 120 mg dose. Adverse events included gastrointestinal (75%), dermatologic (71%), constitutional (68%), pain (64%), and hepatic (61%).

In 2010, George and colleagues undertook a phase II study of regorafenib in patients whose condition had previously failed to respond to both imatinib and sunitinib treatment for GIST [27]. In this trial of 33 patients, an impressive 75% experienced clinical benefit from the use of regorafenib (tumor response of complete or partial response, or stable disease for at least 16 weeks), with an overall PFS for the entire cohort of 10 months (95% CI 8.3–14.9 months). Both patients with wild-type GIST and KIT exon 9 and 11 mutations experienced clinical benefit at comparable rates (no PDGFRA mutations were detected among those in the trial). Those with KIT exon 11 mutations appeared to have a longer PFS compared with those with exon 9 mutations, although numbers were small. Most patients required at least one dose reduction due to toxicity (82%), with the most common adverse events being hand–foot skin reaction, hypertension, fatigue, and diarrhea. A number of these patients were subsequently able to re-escalate their dose of regorafenib. On the basis of the promising results obtained from the phase II study in GIST, the phase III GRID trial was undertaken.

Phase III

The GRID (GIST-regorafenib in progressive disease) trial, a double-blind, placebo-controlled study, enrolled 199 subjects with refractory GIST [10]. This study recruited patients with histologically confirmed, metastatic or unresectable GIST, with failure of at least previous imatinib (either through disease progression or from intolerance) and previous sunitinib (through disease progression only). Patients received regorafenib 160 mg by mouth or placebo daily for 3 out of 4 weeks each cycle.

The primary endpoint of the trial was progression-free survival (PFS) with overall survival (OS) as a secondary endpoint. There was a statistically significant difference between groups for progression-free survival with a median PFS of 4.8 months vs 0.9 months for the regorafenib vs placebo arms, respectively (HR 0.268, 95% CI 0.185–0.388, $P < 0.0001$). Prespecified subgroup analysis demonstrated HR mostly consistent with that of the primary analysis in favor of regorafenib. Specifically, the HR for those with exon 11 and exon 9 mutations were 0.21 (0.10–0.46) and 0.24 (0.07–0.88), respectively. Only the group that were on imatinib less than 6 months had a HR that crossed unity (HR 0.50, 95% CI 0.17–1.73).

There was no difference between groups for overall survival with a hazard ratio (HR) of 0.772 (95% confidence interval [CI]: 0.423, 1.408, *p*-value 0.199). Given the high level of crossover in the trial, the overall survival data should be interpreted with caution. There was no significant difference in benefit achieved between those with exon 9 or exon 11 KIT mutations in this study. Subgroup analysis showed benefit across age groups, geographic location, and line of therapy (third versus fourth line), with only those who had an imatinib duration of less than 6 months failing to show a PFS benefit [28, 29].

9.2.1.4 Safety

The most common adverse reactions reported were HFSR (56%), hypertension (48.5%), diarrhea (40%), and fatigue (38.6%). Of these toxicities less than half were grade 3 or higher. Grade 3 toxicities were seen in 19.7% of HFSR adverse events, 22.7% of hypertension adverse events, 5.3% of diarrhea adverse events, and 2.3% of fatigue adverse events. The only grade 4 toxicity was reported in patients with hypertension with only 0.8% of patients reporting this toxicity.

Severe drug induced liver injury with fatal outcome occurred in 0.3% of 1100 regorafenib-treated patients across all clinical trials. Liver biopsy results, when available, showed hepatocyte necrosis with lymphocyte infiltration. In clinical trial, fatal hepatic failure occurred in 1.6% of patients in the regorafenib arm and 0.4% of patients in the placebo arm; all the patients with hepatic failure had metastatic disease in the liver.

Obtain liver function tests (ALT, AST, and bilirubin) before initiation of regorafenib and monitor at least every 2 weeks during the first 2 months of treatment. Thereafter, monitor monthly or more frequently as clinically indicated. Monitor liver function tests weekly in patients experiencing elevated liver function tests until improvement to less than 3 times the ULN or baseline [30].

Temporarily hold and then reduce or permanently discontinue regorafenib depending on the severity and persistence of hepatotoxicity as manifested by elevated liver function tests or hepatocellular necrosis [31, 32].

9.2.1.5 Mutation Status

A preplanned retrospective biomarker analysis has used the pretreatment tissue specimens from patients enrolled in the GRID trial and compared the mutations detected with those subsequently found in blood samples at the time of resistance to imatinib and sunitinib at the time of entry to GRID. The group found resistance mutations in 48% of the blood samples, but only 12% of the pretreatment tissue samples. In addition, in almost half of those samples that harbored known secondary mutations, multiple mutations were present. Regorafenib showed activity across a range of secondary KIT mutations, reinforcing its utility in this setting, but questions remain about how to differentiate those most likely to respond to treatment from those who will not. In addition, two trials are currently underway, attempting to determine biomarkers that may correlate with clinical efficacy of regorafenib when used for metastatic colorectal cancer. Any positive results from these studies would warrant investigation in the GIST population to determine if the findings were similarly useful and could lead to more judicious use of regorafenib in this group.

References

1. Mendel DB, Laird AD, Xin X, et al. In vivo antitumor activity of SU11248, a novel tyrosine kinase inhibitor targeting vascular endothelial growth factor and platelet-derived growth factor receptors: determination of a pharmacokinetic/pharmacodynamic relationship. Clin Cancer Res. 2003;9(1):327–37.
2. Izzedine H, Buhaescu I, Rixe O, Deray G. Sunitinib malate. Cancer Chemother Pharmacol. 2007;60(3):357–64.

3. Bello CL, Garrett M, Sherman L, Smeraglia J, Ryan B, Toh M. Pharmacokinetics of sunitinib malate in subjects with hepatic impairment. Cancer Chemother Pharmacol. 2010;66(4):699–707.
4. Houk BE, Bello CL, Poland B, Rosen LS, Demetri GD, Motzer RJ. Relationship between exposure to sunitinib and efficacy and tolerability endpoints in patients with cancer: results of a pharmacokinetic/pharmacodynamic meta-analysis. Cancer Chemother Pharmacol. 2010;66(2):357–71.
5. Bello CL, Sherman L, Zhou J, et al. Effect of food on the pharmacokinetics of sunitinib malate (SU11248), a multi-targeted receptor tyrosine kinase inhibitor: results from a phase I study in healthy subjects. Anti-Cancer Drugs. 2006;17(3):353–8.
6. Ikezoe T, Yang Y, Nishioka C, et al. Effect of SU11248 on gastrointestinal stromal tumor-T1 cells: enhancement of growth inhibition via inhibition of 3-kinase/Akt/mammalian target of rapamycin signaling. Cancer Sci. 2006;97(9):945–51.
7. Demetri GD, Heinrich MC, Fletcher JA, et al. Molecular target modulation, imaging, and clinical evaluation of gastrointestinal stromal tumor patients treated with sunitinib malate after imatinib failure. Clin Cancer Res. 2009;15(18):5902–9.
8. Shirao K, Nishida T, Doi T, et al. Phase I/II study of sunitinib malate in Japanese patients with gastrointestinal stromal tumor after failure of prior treatment with imatinib mesylate. Investig New Drugs. 2010;28(6):866–75.
9. Demetri GD, Huang X, Garrett CR, et al. Novel statistical analysis of long-term survival to account for crossover in a phase III trial of sunitinib (SU) vs. placebo (PL) in advanced GIST after imatinib (IM) failure. J Clin Oncol. 2008;26(15S):10524.
10. Demetri GD, Reichardt P, Kang Y-K, et al. Efficacy and safety of regorafenib for advanced gastrointestinal stromal tumors after failure of imatinib and sunitinib (GRID): an international, multicenter, randomized, placebo-controlled, phase 3 trial. Lancet. 2013;381(9863):295–302.
11. Demetri GD, van Oosterom AT, Garrett CR, et al. Efficacy and safety of sunitinib in patients with advanced gastrointestinal stromal tumour after failure of imatinib: a randomized controlled trial. Lancet. 2006;368(9544):1329–38.
12. Demetri GD, Garrett CR, et al. Complete longitudinal analyses of the randomized, placebo-controlled, phase III trial of sunitinib in patients with gastrointestinal stromal tumor following imatinib failure. Clin Cancer Res. 2012;18(11):3170–9.
13. George S, Blay JY, Casali PG, et al. Clinical evaluation of continuous daily dosing of sunitinib malate in patients with advanced gastrointestinal stromal tumour after imatinib failure. Eur J Cancer. 2009;45(11):1959–68.
14. Reichardt P, Kang Y-K, Rutkowski P, et al. Clinical outcomes of patients with advanced gastrointestinal stromal tumors: safety and efficacy in a world- wide treatment-use trial of sunitinib. Cancer. 2015;121(9):1405–13.
15. Lee JL, Kim MK, Park I, et al. Randomized phase II trial of Sunitinib four weeks on and two weeks off versus two weeks on and one week off in metastatic clear-cell type REnal cell carcinoma: RESTORE trial. Ann Oncol. 2015;26(11):2300–5.
16. Bracarda S, Iacovelli R, Boni L, et al. Sunitinib administered on 2/1 schedule in patients with metastatic renal cell carcinoma: the RAINBOW analysis. Ann Oncol. 2015;26(10):2107–13.
17. Khosravan R, Motzer RJ, Fumagalli E, Rini BI. Population pharmacokinetic/pharmacodynamic modeling of sunitinib by dosing schedule in patients with advanced renal cell carcinoma or gastrointestinal stromal tumor. Clin Pharmacokinet. 2016;55(10):1251–69.
18. de Wit D, van Erp NP, Khosravan R, et al. Effect of gastrointestinal resection on sunitinib exposure in patients with GIST. BMC Cancer. 2014;14(1):575.
19. Tielen R, Verhoef C, van Coevorden F, et al. Surgery after treatment with imatinib and/or sunitinib in patients with metastasized gastrointestinal stromal tumors: is it worthwhile? World J Surg Oncol. 2012;10:111.
20. Raut CP, Wang Q, Manola J, et al. Cytoreductive surgery in patients with metastatic gastrointestinal stromal tumor treated with sunitinib malate. Ann Surg Oncol. 2010;17(2):407–15.
21. Nishida T, Takahashi T, Nishitani A, et al. Sunitinib-resistant gastro- intestinal stromal tumors harbor cis-mutations in the activation loop of the KIT gene. Int J Clin Oncol. 2009;14(2):143–9.

22. Rutkowski P, Bylina E, Klimczak A, et al. The outcome and predictive factors of sunitinib therapy in advanced gastrointestinal stromal tumors (GIST) after imatinib failure – one institution study. BMC Cancer. 2012;12(1):107.
23. Heinrich MC, Maki RG, Corless CL, et al. Primary and secondary kinase genotypes correlate with the biological and clinical activity of sunitinib in imatinib-resistant gastrointestinal stromal tumor. J Clin Oncol. 2008;26(33):5352–9.
24. Liegl B, Kepten I, Le C, et al. Heterogeneity of kinase inhibitor resistance mechanisms in GIST. J Pathol. 2008;216(1):64–74.
25. Gajiwala KS, Wu JC, Christensen J, et al. KIT kinase mutants show unique mechanisms of drug resistance to imatinib and sunitinib in gastrointestinal stromal tumor patients. Proc Natl Acad Sci U S A. 2009;106(5):1542–7.
26. Guo T, Hajdu M, Agaram NP, et al. Mechanisms of sunitinib resistance in gastrointestinal stromal tumors harboring KITAY502-3ins mutation: an in vitro mutagenesis screen for drug resistance. Clin Cancer Res. 2009;15(22):6862–70.
27. George S, Wang Q, Heinrich MC, et al. Efficacy and safety of regorafenib in patients with metastatic and/or unresectable GI stromal tumor after failure of imatinib and sunitinib: a multicenter phase II trial. J Clin Oncol. 2012;30(19):2401–7.
28. Casali PG, Reichardt P, Kang Y, et al. Clinical benefit with Regorafenib across subgroups and post-progression in patients with advanced gastrointestinal stromal tumor (Gist) after progression on Imatinib and Sunitinib: phase 3 Grid trial update. Ann Oncol. 2012;23:478–9.
29. Bauer S, Joensuu H, Casali P, et al. Results from a phase III trial (GRID) evaluating regorafenib in metastatic gastrointestinal stromal tumour (GIST): subgroup analysis of outcomes based on pretreatment characteristics. Onkologie. 2013;36:180–1.
30. Blay J, Casali P, Reichardt P, et al. Time course of adverse events in the phase III GRID study of regorafenib in patients with metastatic gastrointestinal stromal tumors (GIST). Eur J Cancer. 2013;49:S884.
31. Reichardt P, Demetri G, Kang YK, et al. Randomized phase 3 trial of regorafenib in patients (pts) with metastatic and/or unresectable gastrointestinal stromal tumor (GIST) progressing despite prior treatment with at least imatinib (IM) and sunitinib (SU)-GRID trial. Onkologie. 2012;35:168.
32. Joensuu H, Casali PG, Reichardt P, et al. Results from a phase III trial (GRID) evaluating regorafenib (REG) in metastatic gastrointestinal stromal tumour (GIST): subgroup analysis of outcomes based on pretreatment characteristics. J Clin Oncol. 2013;31:10551.

Adjuvant and Neoadjuvant Treatment

10

Haruhiko Cho

Abstract

Although surgical complete resection remains the only curative intervention for GIST, more than 40% of completely resected GISTs, especially those expressing high-risk features, such as large tumors or tumors with a high mitotic rate, are likely to develop recurrence with distant metastasis. In the past two decades, tyrosine kinase inhibitors were introduced for the treatment of GIST, and imatinib greatly prolonged the survival of metastatic or unresectable disease. This efficacy has encouraged the use of imatinib in perioperative settings; however, the staging system (risk estimation) is immature, and thus which patients need adjuvant or neoadjuvant therapy the most is unclear. A recent phase III trial revealed that adjuvant imatinib improves the recurrence-free survival of high-risk GISTs, but the optimum duration of imatinib and the impact on the overall survival remain controversial. Neoadjuvant treatment is a promising strategy for marginally resectable GISTs, but the prospective comparison of adjuvant and neoadjuvant therapy for such patients has not been performed. The further accumulation of evidence and the establishment of universal risk estimation and prevalence of genotyping are necessary in order to facilitate the perioperative treatment of GIST.

Keywords

Gastrointestinal stromal tumor · Adjuvant treatment · Neoadjuvant treatment Imatinib

H. Cho (✉)
Department of Surgery, Tokyo Metropolitan Cancer and Infectious Disease Center Komagome Hospital, Tokyo, Japan
e-mail: choharuhiko@cick.jp

Y. Kurokawa, Y. Komatsu (eds.), *Gastrointestinal Stromal Tumor*,
https://doi.org/10.1007/978-981-13-3206-7_10

10.1 Introduction

Gastrointestinal stromal tumors (GISTs) are the most common sarcomas of the gastrointestinal tract. All GISTs are potentially malignant, but their potential ranges from indolent to highly aggressive. Although most localized GISTs are indicative for primary surgery and are completely resected as planned, surgery alone may cause relapse in 40–50% of completely resected GISTs [1, 2].

Approximately, 90% of GISTs harbor gain-of-function mutations in either the KIT or platelet-derived growth factor receptor alpha (PDGFRA) genes [3] that have been identified as driver genes of GIST [4–6]. These mutations are basically mutually exclusive, and different mutations do not exist simultaneously in the same tumor. It can be said that GISTs are a genetically simple and relatively homogeneous disease, except for the so-called wild-type (both KIT/PDGFRA mutation-negative) GISTs, which include several minor mutations, such as NF1 or BRAF. This genetic homogeneity is one of the largest advantages in treating GISTs using tyrosine kinase inhibitors (TKIs).

At present, three TKIs, imatinib, sunitinib, and regorafenib, have been approved as first-, second-, and third-line therapies for the treatment of patients with KIT-positive GISTs. It has been reported that 45–52% of patients with metastatic GIST responded to first-line imatinib with acceptable toxicities [7, 8]. Although surgery remains the mainstay treatment for easily resectable GISTs, surgery alone for locally advanced and/or marginally resectable GISTs is not satisfactory, especially in this era of TKIs.

This review will discuss the significance of the perioperative use of imatinib for localized GISTs.

10.2 Overview

The ultimate goal of perioperative imatinib is to cure locally advanced and/or marginally resectable GISTs in which no residual tumor (R0) is difficult to achieve by surgery alone or in which recurrence may develop even after R0 surgery. As routine lymphadenectomy does not contribute to the outcome of the treatment of GIST, it is also desirable to preserve the organ function and avoid extended surgery as much as possible. However, evidence supporting perioperative adjuvant therapy is insufficient at present, and optimum candidates remain unclear.

10.2.1 Who Benefits from Perioperative Imatinib?

Perioperative therapy includes either or both preoperative or postoperative intervention. Generally, TNM staging is not adapted to the preoperative evaluation of GIST because GISTs rarely metastasize to lymph nodes. The mitotic count is one of the most important factors in evaluating the risk of recurrence; however, its evaluation from a biopsy is not reliable due to the heterogeneity within these tumors [9].

Accordingly, a treatment decision is made by not only pathological findings but also by considering the clinically specific features of GIST, such as tumor rupture.

10.2.1.1 Large GISTs

Patients with GISTs rarely complain of symptoms associated with bowel obstruction because large GISTs usually develop expansively and extraluminally. Almost two-thirds of patients with GIST had tumors over 5 cm in size at the diagnosis, and some tumors grew to be as large as 40 cm [1]. The tumor volume doubling time on computed tomography (CT) was reported to be almost 1 year [10], which is significantly shorter than schwannoma (doubling time: 4.6 years). This rapid growth without symptoms may allow these tumors to grow large, making complete resection difficult.

In general, the complete resection rates for GISTs without metastasis are reported to be around 80% by surgery alone [2]. Even after the tumor is completely resected, large GISTs still have considerably high risks of recurrence. The 5-year recurrence-free survival (RFS) rate of large GIST (>10 cm) is 35–50% if the patient does not receive adjuvant therapy [1]. Neoadjuvant treatment is a promising strategy for large GISTs with low complete resection rates and a high risk of rupture. In addition, in tumors >10 cm in size, downstaging (to a lower-risk category) does not occur only by pathological modification from neoadjuvant treatment because "size >10 cm" is itself a definitive factor for the high-risk category.

10.2.1.2 Tumors with Rupture or at Risk of Rupture

At tumor rupture, tumor cells spill and become disseminated in the abdominal cavity. Therefore, macroscopic complete resection of ruptured GIST is treated as R1 surgery, not as R0. The prognosis of ruptured GIST is poor; the 5-year RFS rate of ruptured GIST is approximately 20% if the patient does not receive adjuvant therapy [1]. Ruptured GISTs have a high risk for peritoneal recurrence in theory, but more exactly, preoperative spontaneous rupture and intraoperative rupture associated with surgical manipulation should be differently classified because the intraoperatively disseminated tumor cells could be washed and collected before they are implanted in the peritoneum.

Tumor rupture occurs in 5–7% of GISTs [1, 11] and does not always happen to large GISTs. In a study of 23 patients with ruptured GISTs [12], the median tumor size of the ruptured lesions was 8 cm (range 4–28 cm). The association between the tumor growth pattern and the occurrence of peritoneal metastasis was examined in another study. It was reported that peritoneal metastasis more frequently occurred in extraluminal tumors (50%: 15/30) than in intraluminal tumors (10%: 1/10) [13]. Although whether or not tumor shrinkage due to imatinib prevents spontaneous tumor rupture is unclear, tumor rupture during imatinib treatment in neoadjuvant setting has not been reported.

10.2.1.3 Difficult-to-Resect Anatomical Location

GISTs can arise from all digestive tracts, with frequencies of 5% in esophagus, 70% in stomach, 20% in small intestine, and 5% in colon and rectum. Among these sites, the esophagus, duodenum, and rectum are located in the narrow spaces of the mediastinum, retroperitoneum, and pelvis, respectively. Tumors occurring in these sites are difficult to resect and likely to rupture during surgery, and preserving the organ function is also difficult. Tumor shrinkage may improve the surgical difficulty and prevent intraoperative tumor rupture, and it may also help avoid highly invasive surgery, e.g., pancreaticoduodenectomy (PD) in duodenal GIST and rectal amputation in rectal GIST. It was reported that 30–40% of patients with duodenal GIST underwent PD, and the rest underwent conservative surgery, but the surgical approach did not affect the risk of recurrence [14, 15].

10.2.1.4 "High-Risk" GISTs

The term "high-risk" refers to patients who have been clinically or pathologically evaluated as being at high risk for recurrence after macroscopic complete surgery (R0 or R1). Several risk factors for recurrence in GIST were identified, and which of these is the strongest prognosticator has been the subject of some debate. Four factors are now widely accepted as predictive factors of recurrence: the mitotic count, tumor size, tumor site, and rupture. Originally, the risk for each tumor was evaluated by the combination of two factors (mitotic count and tumor size) under the National Institute of Health (NIH) consensus criteria [16]. Thereafter, primary site was added in the Armed Forces Institute of Pathology (AFIP) criteria [17], and tumor rupture was added in the modified NIH consensus criteria [18]. The 5-year RFS rate of high-risk GISTs under the modified NIH consensus criteria is around 40% if the patient does not receive adjuvant therapy [1]. Patients evaluated as high-risk before operation are candidates for both adjuvant and neoadjuvant therapy (Fig. 10.1).

10.2.1.5 Imatinib-Sensitive GIST

Tumor genotyping is a predictive marker of the efficacy of imatinib, and most of the mutational subtypes in GIST respond well to imatinib. Several subtypes (PDGFRA exon18 D842V, KIT exon17 D816V, and both KIT/PDGFRA wild-type) are known to have no or an inferior response to imatinib [19]. KIT exon9 has a higher response to high-dose (800 mg/day) than to low-dose (400 mg/day) imatinib [20], but high-dose imatinib is not approved for GIST in Japan. Therefore, patients with such imatinib-resistant mutations are at risk of receiving ineffective treatment for a long time if they receive adjuvant treatment and may miss the chance to undergo surgery due to tumor progression if they receive neoadjuvant treatment.

10.3 Adjuvant Therapy

In the setting of advanced and metastatic GISTs, a longer survival has been shown to be correlated more closely with smaller tumors in the treatment of imatinib than with larger tumors. If imatinib responds in reverse proportion to the tumor size, then microscopic metastasis would be the best target of imatinib therapy in theory. However, the standard method for detecting microscopic metastasis has not yet been established.

The target patients who warrant adjuvant imatinib are currently being discussed in terms of the tumor stage (risk estimation) and sensitivity to imatinib (genotyping). As with other sarcoma tumors, GISTs are proposed to obey a classification system defined by tumor size and pathological grade. This is called "risk classification" or "risk criteria." Under the original NIH consensus criteria, the mitotic count per 50 high-power fields (HPF) was used as the index for the pathological grade. The survival curves of each risk group classified by the NIH consensus criteria are clearly separated, but some problems may arise when the original NIH consensus criteria is used for selecting optimum patients who would benefit from adjuvant therapy with imatinib.

The first problem is the issue of discontinuity of risk. Since both the tumor size and mitotic count are continuous variables, the risk of a tumor is likely to be evaluated differently if there is even a small difference in the tumor size or mitotic count around the cut-off value. For example, a 5.0-cm GIST with a mitotic count of 5/50 HPF is evaluated as a low-risk lesion, but a 5.1-cm GIST with a mitotic count of 6/50HPF is evaluated as a high-risk lesion. For such marginal cases, the supplemental usage of another tool is recommended. Contour maps for predicting the 10-year risk of recurrence after surgery are useful for reducing this gap in risk estimation [1].

The second problem is the issue of the reliability and reproducibility of the mitotic count. The criteria for identifying mitosis are different between pathologists [21]. Indeed, the mitotic count is reported to differ between local and central pathologists. In general, local pathologists tend to count mitosis higher than central pathologists. The field-of-view of the eyepiece for the microscope should also be noted. The field-of-view of more recently manufactured eyepieces is almost twice that of older eyepieces. The European Society for Medical Oncology (ESMO) guideline recommends that the mitotic count be expressed as the number in a 5-mm^2 area, which is equivalent to 50 HPFs with a conventional eyepiece [22]. Other methods like the Ki-67 labeling index have also been considered for use in place of the mitotic count, although the mitotic count has yet to be replaced formally.

10.3.1 Clinical Trials

To date, two phase I and three phase II trials of adjuvant therapy have been conducted. The results have already been published, excluding one phase II trial (PERSIST5). All of these trials have targeted "high-risk" GISTs, but the definition of high-risk varied among trials (Table 10.1). Whether or not adjuvant therapy should target intermediate-risk patients under the NIH consensus criteria as well as high-risk patients is still controversial. No trial has yet mandated genotyping before registration.

10.3.1.1 ACOSOG Z9000

Based on the successful results of imatinib for advanced or metastatic GIST, the first phase II trial, ACOSOG Z9000, was conducted to test the efficacy and safety of adjuvant imatinib [23]. A total of 106 patients were accrued, and the patients were

Table 10.1 Differences of eligibility criteria in phase II/III trial of adjuvant imatinib

Trial	Phase	Intervention	Inclusion criteria (tumor)
ACOSOG Z9000	II	Imatinib 400 mg/day for 12M	Size >10 cm, tumor rupture, peritoneal implants (up to 4)
PERCIST5	II	Imatinib 400 mg/day for 60M	Primary GIST (any site): ≥ 2 cm and a mitotic rate of ≥ 5/50 HPFs Non-gastric primary GIST: ≥ 5 cm
ACOSOG Z9001	III	Placebo vs Imatinib 400 mg/day for 12M	Size ≥3 cm
SSG-XVIII	III	Imatinib 400 mg/day for 12M vs for 36M	High risk at NIH consensus criteria or tumor rupture
EORTC62024	III	Placebo vs Imatinib 400 mg/day for 24M	High and intermediate risk at NIH consensus criteria

prescribed imatinib 400 mg/day for 1 year. The primary endpoint was the overall survival (OS), and adjuvant imatinib was expected to prolong the OS from 35% (historical control) to 50%. The secondary endpoints were the RFS and patient safety. The 5-year OS rate was 83%, which was more favorable than expected. The 1-, 3-, and 5-year RFS rates were 96%, 60%, and 40%. Although adjuvant imatinib prevented recurrence in most cases, the effect did not continue after the termination of treatment. The median RFS of the patients with KIT exon11 was more favorable than that of those with KIT exon9 (42 vs. 19 months) but poorer than that of those with PDGFRA and wild-type. The result was consistent with the data reported in a previous trial of advanced and metastatic settings. The finding that none of the patients with KIT exon9 recurred in the first year indicated that imatinib 400 mg/day is effective for the prevention of recurrence even in patients with KIT exon9. Although high-dose (800 mg/day) imatinib was associated with a longer survival among patients with the KIT exon9 mutation in the advanced and metastatic settings, whether or not high-dose imatinib has a more favorable effect than low-dose administration in an adjuvant setting is unclear.

10.3.1.2 ACOSOG Z9001

The ACOSOG Z9001 is a randomized phase III, double-blind trial [24]. A total of 713 patients who had a histological diagnosis of primary GIST measuring ≥3 cm in size were randomly assigned to receive 1 year of adjuvant imatinib at a dose of 400 mg/day or 1 year of placebo. The original primary endpoint was the OS, which was then changed to the RFS because it gradually became clear that the event (death) rarely occurred if patients received imatinib therapy after recurrence. The trial was stopped early following the planned interim analysis because significantly fewer patients experienced recurrence with the drug than with the placebo. These findings indicated that 1-year imatinib did indeed significantly improve the RFS compared with placebo, with an RFS rate at 1 year of 98% in the imatinib group and 83% in the placebo group and a hazard ratio of 0.35 (95% confidence interval: 0.22–0.53). In risk factor analysis, a large tumor size (>10 cm), high mitotic count (≥10/50 HPF), and small bowel origin were independent risk factors for a worse

RFS in imatinib arm as well as placebo arm [25]. Strangely, the hazard ratio of large tumor size (>10 cm) against reference (size <5 cm) in imatinib arm was 6.51, and it was rather increased as compared with the hazard ratio in placebo arm (3.25). This result might suggest that the benefit of adjuvant imatinib was smaller in large GIST than in small GIST, and another strategy should be considered for large GISTs. The RFS for patients with KIT exon11 was longer in the imatinib group than in the placebo group. The same trend was not observed in patients with KIT exon9 and wild-type tumors.

10.3.1.3 EORTC62024

The EORTC62024 trial was a randomized phase III trial comparing 2 years of adjuvant imatinib to observation alone [26]. The original primary endpoint was the OS but was changed to imatinib failure-free survival (IFFS) in 2009, given the recent development of post-imatinib treatment and improvement in the prognosis. The IFFS was defined as the time to death or starting another TKI. A total of 908 patients were randomly assigned to adjuvant imatinib or observation. The patients who had high-risk tumors (i.e., mitotic count >10/50 HPF and tumor diameter over 10 cm, or mitotic count >5/50 HPF and a tumor diameter of over 5 cm) or intermediate-risk tumors (i.e., tumor size ≤5 cm and mitotic count 6/50 to 10/50 HPF, or tumor size >5 to 10 cm and mitotic count ≤5/50 HPF) were eligible. Briefly, there was a significant difference in the RFS (84% in the imatinib arm and 64% in the observation arm at 3 years, log-rank $p < 0.001$), but no significant difference in the 5-year IFFS (87% in the imatinib arm and 84% in the observation arm, hazard ratio [HR]: 0.79, 98.5% CI of 0.50–1.25). When the analysis of the 5-year IFFS was limited only to the high-risk subcategory, there was a trend favoring the imatinib arm, but it was not statistically significant (79% in the imatinib arm and 73% in the observation arm, $p = 0.087$).

10.3.1.4 SSG XVIII

A phase III randomized controlled trial conducted by the Scandinavian Sarcoma Group (SSG) compared 36 months vs. 12 months of adjuvant imatinib after the resection of high-risk GIST [27]. The eligibility criteria of this study were one of the following: mitotic count >10/50 HPF and tumor diameter >10 cm, mitotic count >5/50 HPF and tumor diameter >5 cm, or tumor rupture. The tumor site was not considered for the high-risk definition. A total of 400 patients were allocated to each group. A central pathological review confirmed that 15 of 397 patients (4%) were not GIST. At a median follow-up of 54 months, the 5-year RFS was significantly longer in the 36-month group than in the 12-month group (65.6% vs. 47.9%, HR = 0.46 with 95% CI of 0.32–0.65, $P < 0.001$). Furthermore, the 5-year OS was also significantly longer in the 36-month group than in the 12-month group (92.0% vs. 81.7%, HR = 0.45 with 95% CI, 0.22–0.89; $P = 0.02$). The second planned analysis at a median follow-up of 90 months revealed that the survival benefit persisted with a longer 5-year RFS (71.1% vs. 52.3%) and 5-year OS (91.9% vs. 85.3%) in the 36-month group compared with the 12-month group [28]. Adverse events occurred more frequently in the 36-month group than in the 12-month group, but the grade was generally mild. The most common event in the 36-month group was anemia (80.3%), followed by periorbital edema (74.2%) and diarrhea (54%). Adverse events were associated with treatment discontinuation in 13.6% of the 36-month group and 7.5% of the 12-month group.

10.3.2 Patient Selection

There is rough consensus among experts that risk estimation tools should be used for optimum patient selection for adjuvant therapy; however, which tool should be used and what cut-off should be selected remain unclear. Joensuu et al. [1] compared the prognostic accuracy of risk estimation tools using a receiver operating characteristic (ROC) curve and found in estimating the 10-year recurrence risk that the best predictor of recurrence was a nonlinear model that included tumor rupture data. The areas under the curve (AUCs) of the nonlinear model including rupture, the NIH consensus criteria, AFIP criteria, and modified NIH consensus criteria were 0.88, 0.79, 0.82, and 0.78, respectively. These analyses suggested that it is better to use a tool that includes tumor rupture when adjuvant therapy is considered, although the definition of tumor rupture remains unclear. The indication for adjuvant therapy should be carefully considered for patients who suffer from tumor rupture as a single high-risk factor.

As for the cut-off of risk category, that for high-risk is definite, but that for intermediate-risk is controversial. In the EORTC62024 study, which included intermediate-risk patients in their eligibility criteria, there were no statistically significant differences in the RFS between the high- and intermediate-risk subgroups ($p = 0.111$). At present, data are insufficient to determine whether or not patients with intermediate risk benefit from adjuvant imatinib. We should at least not include all patients with intermediate risk and instead screen patients or reevaluate individual risk using several risk estimation tools (please refer to Chap. 5).

10.3.3 Optimum Duration of Adjuvant Therapy

The ideal goal of adjuvant therapy is the complete elimination of minimal residual disease and cure. Generally, the duration of adjuvant therapy is about 6 months to 1 year in gastrointestinal cancers, such as gastric cancer or colorectal cancer. GISTs also occur from the digestive tract, but the duration of adjuvant therapy is considered differently from gastrointestinal cancers because imatinib acts as a cytostatic agent rather than a cytotoxic agent.

Whether the long-term treatment of imatinib can eradicate microscopic disease or simply delays recurrence is controversial. Two conflicting results have been found concerning the effect of adjuvant imatinib. In the SSG XVIII trial, a longer treatment (3 years) improved not only the RFS but also the OS compared with a shorter treatment (1 year). In contrast, in the EORTC62024 study, 2 years of adjuvant imatinib helped prolong the RFS but did not prolong the OS compared to observation alone.

Determining which evidence is more appropriate to extrapolate to clinical practice is difficult because of several differences between the two studies. For example, patients with intermediate risk were included in the EORTC study but not in the Scandinavian study. In addition, the standard arm was observation alone in the EORTC study but 1-year imatinib in the Scandinavian study. Furthermore, the duration of adjuvant imatinib in the test arm was also different, being 2 years in the EORTC study and 3 years in the Scandinavian study. We also have little information on post-imatinib treatment, which may have a large impact on the OS.

Despite these differences, a longer duration of imatinib was associated with a longer RFS in both studies. The effect of further long duration of imatinib (5 years) is currently being evaluated in the PERSIST5 study.

In summary, 2–3 years of adjuvant imatinib is acceptable and can be recommended for maintaining a long RFS. The follow-up and post-imatinib therapy as well as the duration of adjuvant therapy are important for prolonging the OS.

10.3.4 Follow-Up After Stopping Adjuvant Therapy

As adjuvant imatinib reduces the risk of recurrence after surgery, the patients who underwent adjuvant imatinib might as well follow the modified examination schedule of high-risk GIST. During the adjuvant period, the risk of recurrence is small, unless the patient has a tumor with an imatinib-resistant genotype. The ESMO guideline describes a routine follow-up schedule for patients with GIST who undergo adjuvant therapy, and a follow-up example with an imaging interval of every 3–6 months during adjuvant therapy is mentioned [22]. Patients with an unavailable tumor genotype are recommended to receive a checkup every 3 months. After discontinuation of adjuvant imatinib, the risk of recurrence is likely to increase. In the SSG XVIII trial, recurrence frequently occurred after stopping adjuvant imatinib in both the 1-year and 3-year arms. Therefore, patients who undergo adjuvant imatinib should receive follow-up with a short interval including imaging examinations every 3 months for 2 years after stopping adjuvant therapy. Thereafter, once in every 6 months for several years is a feasible interval for imaging examinations.

10.4 Neoadjuvant Therapy

Complete surgical resection is the only curative intervention for GIST; however, the resectability is marginal when the tumor has at least one of the following: large size, origin at a difficult-to-resect anatomical location, or risk of rupture. The success of imatinib in the advanced and metastatic settings has supported its use in the neoadjuvant setting for locally advanced or marginally resectable GISTs. In particular, the high response rate and tumor-associated shrinkage suggested benefits with this agent in preoperative treatment.

In the phase II study of imatinib 400 mg/day for unresectable or metastatic GIST, the overall response rate was 68.5% (complete response [CR]: 0%, and partial response [PR]: 68.5%) in the lower-dose group [29]. In another retrospective study, imatinib reduced the tumor diameter and tumor volume by 43% and 83% at the timing of best response [30]. Volume reduction may help prevent intraoperative tumor rupture, especially in the narrow regions of the mediastinum, retroperitoneum, and pelvis. The potential advantages of neoadjuvant imatinib are facilitating complete resection and preventing extended surgery as well as recurrence after surgery. In addition, evaluating the response to preoperative treatment by imaging provides useful information for postoperative therapy in which no target lesion is available. However, CR is associated with a loss of pathological information. RECIST CR is very rare in GIST, but we sometimes experience cases in which tumor cells are almost completely absent and no mitosis is observed. As the risk estimation of GIST largely depends on pathological findings, it then becomes difficult to evaluate the risk of recurrence correctly in such cases. Information on the genotype is also likely to be lost unless the genotype has already been analyzed using biopsy tissue.

10.4.1 Clinical Trials

At present, the results of two phase II studies of neoadjuvant imatinib for GIST are available (Table 10.2). The results of another trial (APOLLON study) remain unpublished.

10.4.1.1 RTOG0132

The radiation therapy oncology group (RTOG) 0132 was a prospective phase II study to evaluate the efficacy and safety of neoadjuvant imatinib [31]. The initial dose of imatinib was 600 mg/day. Patients with primary GIST (size ≥5 cm) or recurrent/metastatic tumor (≥2 cm) were eligible. The clinical endpoints were the OS, PFS, time to progression (TTP), response (RECIST), toxicity, and surgical complications. A total of 63 patients (30 primary and 22 metastatic) were ultimately enrolled in the study and received preoperative imatinib therapy for 8–12 weeks and postoperative imatinib for 2 years. Imatinib was stopped on the day before surgery and resumed as soon as possible postoperatively.

Table 10.2 Efficacy of neoadjuvant study

	Phase	Intervention	R0 resection rate	Survival
RTOG0132	II	Imatinib 600 mg/day for 8–12W	77% (primary disease group)	2-year OS rate: 93%
				2-year PFS rate: 83%
Asian trial	II	Imatinib 400 mg/day for 6–9M	91%	2-year OS rate: 98%
				2-year RFS rate: 89%

In the primary tumor group, tumors mildly responded to preoperative imatinib (PR in 7% and stable disease in 83% by RECIST), with no cases of CR or progressive disease during the neoadjuvant period. In contrast, 36 of 44 (81.8%) patients had a complete or partial metabolic response at 1 week on fluorodeoxyglucose-positron emission tomography (FDG-PET) [32]. The mean SUVmax decreased from 14.2 (baseline) to 5.5 (at 1 week). There was one anastomotic disruption. An updated result at a median follow-up of 5.1 years revealed the 5-year PFS and 5-year OS of all patients to be 46.1% and 73.6%, respectively. A high proportion of patients experienced disease progression after termination of 2-year postoperative imatinib therapy [33].

10.4.1.2 Asian Phase II for Large Gastric GIST

An Asian multinational phase II study for patients with gastric GISTs ≥10 cm was conducted to investigate the efficacy and safety of neoadjuvant imatinib [34]. The sample size was calculated based on the hypothesis that neoadjuvant imatinib would improve the R0 resection rate from 70% (historical control) to 85%. The primary endpoint was the R0 resection rate. A total of 56 patients were enrolled in this study and received neoadjuvant imatinib (400 mg/day) for 6–9 months. Neoadjuvant imatinib for ≥6 months was completed in 46 patients. The response rate by RECIST was 62% (95% CI, 48–75%), and median shrinkage rate was 35.4% (range, 0.0–87.0%) (Fig. 10.1). Interestingly, two patients with wild-type GIST responded to neoadjuvant imatinib with rather high shrinkage rate (40.8% and 50.5%). Toxicities were generally mild and there were no treatment-related deaths. The R0 resection rate was 91% (48/53; 95% CI, 79–97%), and organ preservation was achieved in 42 of 48 patients with R0 resection. The 2-year overall and progression-free survival rates were 98% and 89% at a median follow-up time of 32 months.

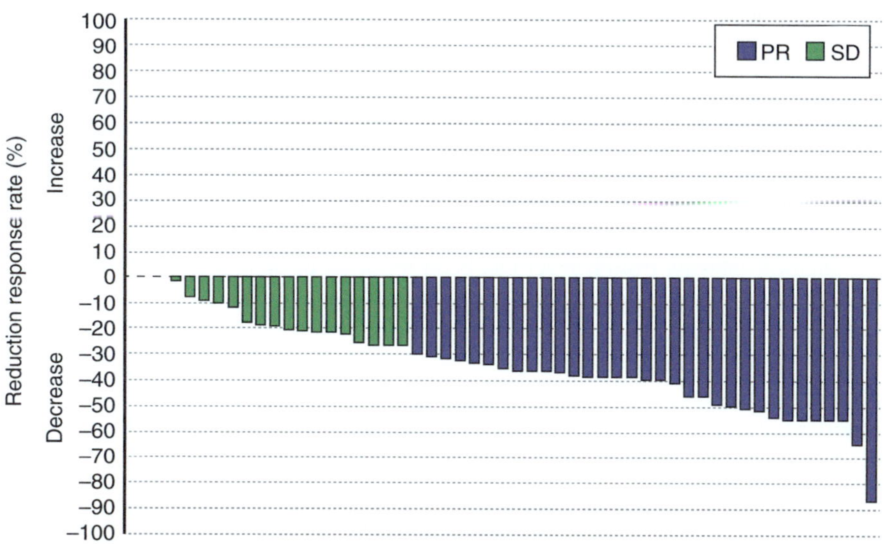

Fig. 10.1 Waterfall plot of tumor shrinkage after neoadjuvant imatinib in Asian phase II study [34]

10.4.2 Duration of Imatinib in Neoadjuvant Therapy

From the perspective of surgical difficulty, it is preferable that tumors be as small as possible, so the preoperative duration of imatinib should be set to reduce the tumor size as much as possible in the neoadjuvant setting. However, the time to best response differs among patients. In the B2222 randomized phase II trial, the median time to response was 2.7 months (range 0.8–39 months), and the time to 75% achieving response was 5.3 months [29]. The median PFS was 24 months (95% CI: 17–30 months). In another phase III study (EORTC62005) in the metastatic setting, the median time to best response was 107 days (interquartile range [IQR]: 58–172 days) [8].

Also in a neoadjuvant setting, the radiologic assessment of the best and plateau response has been reported. In a retrospective study, 20 patients underwent neoadjuvant imatinib with a median treatment duration of 32 weeks. The median time to earliest PR was 16 weeks (IQR 7–26 weeks), and the median time to best response was 28 weeks (IQR18–37 weeks). The time to plateau response was 34 weeks (IQR 24–41 weeks). The tumor size and location did not correlate with the time to best response. Indeed, a short duration of treatment was not effective in the RTOG0132 study. The PR rate was only 7%, and 32% of all nonmetastatic group were unable to achieve complete resection. In contrast, a longer duration was associated with a high R0 resection rate (91%) in the Asian phase II study.

From these data, approximately 6 months (up to 1 year) is reasonable and feasible for achieving adequate tumor shrinkage. Further treatment may increase the risk of imatinib resistance. Imatinib can be continued up to the day before surgery if there is no sign of intestinal edema or severe hematological toxicity. Regarding the timing of starting imatinib after surgery, it is recommended that treatment be started as soon as possible when the patient can take food orally. A consensus-based recommendation supports a total of 3 years of adjuvant imatinib (including preoperative period) based on the results of SSG XVIII.

10.4.3 Operative Procedure

The imatinib plasma trough level has been reported to be associated with the survival in the treatment of GIST, and it was lower in patients with major gastrectomy (942 ± 330 ng/mL) than in those without major gastrectomy (1393 ± 659 ng/mL) [35]. Furthermore, major gastrectomy was found to be an independent risk factor of a lower trough level of plasma imatinib [36]. Therefore, organ preservation is important, especially in patients scheduled to receive postoperative imatinib therapy. Neoadjuvant imatinib is expected to help preserve the organ function through tumor shrinkage.

10.5 Future Directions

No technique has yet been developed to identify microscopic minimal metastasis of GIST. Therefore, no alternative method has been proposed for selecting the best patients to receive adjuvant therapy other than predicting patients who are at a significantly high risk for recurrence. Recently, free-circulating DNA (fcDNA), which is probably released by apoptotic or necrotic tumor cells, has been reported to be a promising marker in patients with tumors and suggests the existence of minimal metastasis or minimal residual disease after curative surgery. In the study of fcDNA in GIST, it was reported that a low level of fcDNA carrying mutations for KIT or PDGFRA was detected in 35% (6/17) of postsurgical patients who had a high or intermediate risk for recurrence [37]. Although the number of patients in the study was too small to draw any hard conclusions and the association between the risk of recurrence and positivity of fcDNA is still unclear, these findings suggest that the detection of fcDNA might be useful for identifying those patients who will most benefit from postoperative adjuvant therapy in the future.

Which patients will most benefit from adjuvant or neoadjuvant therapy remains unclear, and the indication of adjuvant therapy partially overlaps with that of neoadjuvant therapy. When a tumor is larger than 10 cm, the neoadjuvant approach is preferable, irrespective of tumor location, as such tumors are likely to rupture and invade other organs. When the tumor size is 5–10 cm, upfront surgery is recommended, because the recurrence risk should be precisely estimated before the pathological findings are degenerated by imatinib. However, the Japanese guideline states that tumors larger than 5 cm are not suitable for laparoscopic resection. I therefore hypothesize that the risk of intraoperative rupture may be decreased if the tumor size can be reduced to <5 cm. As the median tumor shrinkage rate is reported to be around 40% by neoadjuvant imatinib for 6 months, tumors up to 8 cm in size should decrease to <5 cm with upfront imatinib, in theory. I speculate that GISTs larger than 5 cm, but smaller than 8 cm, are future candidates for clinical trials to verify the efficacy and safety of neoadjuvant imatinib followed by laparoscopic surgery.

10.6 Conclusion

The standard of care for patients with localized GIST is surgery, but a multidisciplinary approach is essential for obtaining further improvements in patient survival. Based on the results of the SSG XVIII trial and EORTC 62024 trial, 2–3 years of adjuvant imatinib after complete resection can be recommended for imatinib-sensitive high-risk GIST in order to maintain a long RFS. Another promising approach is neoadjuvant therapy, and a recent phase II trial of neoadjuvant imatinib demonstrated a favorable survival, high R0 resection rate, and high organ preservation rate in a limited patient group. Although these findings are early ones and the Japanese guideline does not recommend routine practical use, the case-by-case introduction of neoadjuvant imatinib is feasible when a tumor is marginally resectable and harbors an imatinib-sensitive genotype.

References

1. Joensuu H, Vehtari A, Riihimäki J, Nishida T, Steigen SE, Brabec P, et al. Risk of recurrence of gastrointestinal stromal tumour after surgery: an analysis of pooled population-based cohorts. Lancet Oncol. 2012;13:265–74.
2. DeMatteo RP, Lewis JJ, Leung D, Mudan SS, Woodruff JM, Brennan MF. Two hundred gastrointestinal stromal tumors: recurrence patterns and prognostic factors for survival. Ann Surg. 2000;231:51–8.
3. Rubin BP, Heinrich MC, Corless CL. Gastrointestinal stromal tumour. Lancet. 2007;369:1731–41.
4. Hirota S, Isozaki K, Moriyama Y, Hashimoto K, Nishida T, Ishiguro S, et al. Gain-of-function mutations of c-kit in human gastrointestinal stromal tumors. Science. 1998;279:577–80.
5. Heinrich MC, Corless CL, Duensing A, McGreevey L, Chen CJ, Joseph N, et al. PDGFRA activating mutations in gastrointestinal stromal tumors. Science. 2003;299:708–10.
6. Hirota S, Ohashi A, Nishida T, Isozaki K, Kinoshita K, Shinomura Y, et al. Gain-of-function mutations of platelet-derived growth factor receptor alpha gene in gastrointestinal stromal tumors. Gastroenterology. 2003;125:660–7.
7. Blanke CD, Rankin C, Demetri GD, Ryan CW, von Mehren M, Benjamin RS, et al. Phase III randomized, intergroup trial assessing imatinib mesylate at two dose levels in patients with unresectable or metastatic gastrointestinal stromal tumors expressing the kit receptor tyrosine kinase: S0033. J Clin Oncol. 2008;26:626–32.
8. Verweij J, Casali PG, Zalcberg J, LeCesne A, Reichardt P, Blay JY, et al. Progression-free survival in gastrointestinal stromal tumours with high-dose imatinib: randomised trial. Lancet. 2004;364:1127–34.
9. Ricci R, Chiarello G, Attili F, Fuccio L, Alfieri S, Persiani R, et al. Endoscopic ultrasound-guided fine needle tissue acquisition biopsy samples do not allow a reliable proliferation assessment of gastrointestinal stromal tumours. Dig Liver Dis. 2015;47:291–5.
10. Choi JW, Choi D, Kim KM, Sohn TS, Lee JH, Kim HJ, et al. Small submucosal tumors of the stomach: differentiation of gastric schwannoma from gastrointestinal stromal tumor with CT. Korean J Radiol. 2012;13:425–33.
11. Rutkowski P, Bylina E, Wozniak A, Nowecki ZI, Osuch C, Matlok M, et al. Validation of the Joensuu risk criteria for primary resectable gastrointestinal stromal tumour – the impact of tumour rupture on patient outcomes. Eur J Surg Oncol. 2011;37:890–6.
12. Hohenberger P, Ronellenfitsch U, Oladeji O, Pink D, Ströbel P, Wardelmann E, et al. Pattern of recurrence in patients with ruptured primary gastrointestinal stromal tumour. Br J Surg. 2010;97:1854–9.
13. Agaimy A, Vassos N, Wunsch PH, Hohenberger W, Hartmann A, Croner RS. Impact of serosal involvement/extramural growth on the risk of synchronous and metachronous peritoneal spread in gastrointestinal stromal tumors: proposal for a macroscopic classification of GIST. Int J Clin Exp Pathol. 2012;5:12–22.
14. Tien YW, Lee CY, Huang CC, Hu RH, Lee PH. Surgery for gastrointestinal stromal tumors of the duodenum. Ann Surg Oncol. 2010;17:109–14.
15. Johnston FM, Kneuertz PJ, Cameron JL, Sanford D, Fisher S, Turley R, et al. Presentation and management of gastrointestinal stromal tumors of the duodenum: a multi-institutional analysis. Ann Surg Oncol. 2012;19:3351–60.

16. Fletcher CD, Berman JJ, Corless C, Gorstein F, Lasota J, Longley BJ, et al. Diagnosis of gastrointestinal stromal tumors: a consensus approach. Int J Surg Pathol. 2002;10:81–9.
17. Miettinen M, Lasota J. Gastrointestinal stromal tumors: pathology and prognosis at different sites. Semin Diagn Pathol. 2006;23:70–83.
18. Joensuu H. Risk stratification of patients diagnosed with gastrointestinal stromal tumor. Hum Pathol. 2008;39:1411–9.
19. Nishida T, Blay JY, Hirota S, Kitagawa Y, Kang YK. The standard diagnosis, treatment, and follow-up of gastrointestinal stromal tumors based on guidelines. Gastric Cancer. 2016;19(1):3–14.
20. Heinrich MC, Owzar K, Corless CL, Hollis D, Borden EC, Fletcher CD, et al. Correlation of kinase genotype and clinical outcome in the North American Intergroup Phase III Trial of imatinib mesylate for treatment of advanced gastrointestinal stromal tumor: CALGB 150105 study by Cancer and Leukemia Group B and Southwest Oncology Group. J Clin Oncol. 2008;26:5360–7.
21. Ray-Coquard I, Montesco MC, Coindre JM, Dei Tos AP, Lurkin A, Ranchère-Vince D, et al. Sarcoma: concordance between initial diagnosis and centralized expert review in a population-based study within three European regions. Ann Oncol. 2012;23:2442–9.
22. ESMO/European Sarcoma Network Working Group. Gastrointestinal stromal tumors: ESMO Clinical Practice Guidelines for diagnosis, treatment and follow-up. Ann Oncol. 2012;23(Suppl 7). vii49–55.
23. DeMatteo RP, Ballman KV, Antonescu CR, Corless C, Kolesnikova V, von Mehren M, et al. Long-term results of adjuvant imatinib mesylate in localized, high-risk, primary gastrointestinal stromal tumor: ACOSOG Z9000 (Alliance) intergroup phase 2 trial. Ann Surg. 2013;258:422–9.
24. Dematteo RP, Ballman KV, Antonescu CR, Maki RG, Pisters PW, Demetri GD, et al. Adjuvant imatinib mesylate after resection of localised, primary gastrointestinal stromal tumour: a randomised, double-blind, placebo-controlled trial. Lancet. 2009;373:1097–104.
25. Corless CL, Ballman KV, Antonescu CR, Kolesnikova V, Maki RG, Pisters PW, et al. Pathologic and molecular features correlate with long-term outcome after adjuvant therapy of resected primary GI stromal tumor: the ACOSOG Z9001 trial. J Clin Oncol. 2014;32: 1563–70.
26. Casali PG, Le Cesne A, Poveda Velasco A, Kotasek D, Rutkowski P, et al. Time to definitive failure to the first tyrosine kinase inhibitor in localized GI stromal tumors treated with imatinib as an adjuvant: a European Organisation for Research and Treatment of Cancer Soft Tissue and Bone Sarcoma Group Intergroup Randomized Trial in Collaboration with the Australasian Gastro-Intestinal Trials Group, UNICANCER, French Sarcoma Group, Italian Sarcoma Group, and Spanish Group for Research on Sarcomas. J Clin Oncol. 2015;33:4276–83.
27. Joensuu H, Eriksson M, Sundby Hall K, Hartmann JT, Pink D, Schütte J, et al. One vs three years of adjuvant imatinib for operable gastrointestinal stromal tumor: a randomized trial. JAMA. 2012;307:1265–72.
28. Joensuu H, Eriksson M, Sundby Hall K, Reichardt A, Hartmann JT, Pink D, et al. Adjuvant imatinib for high-risk GI stromal tumor: analysis of a randomized trial. J Clin Oncol. 2016;34:244–50.
29. Blanke CD, Demetri GD, von Mehren M, Heinrich MC, Eisenberg B, Fletcher JA, et al. Long-term results from a randomized phase II trial of standard- versus higher-dose imatinib mesylate for patients with unresectable or metastatic gastrointestinal stromal tumors expressing KIT. J Clin Oncol. 2008;26:620–5.
30. Tirumani SH, Shinagare AB, Jagannathan JP, Krajewski KM, Ramaiya NH, Raut CP. Radiologic assessment of earliest, best, and plateau response of gastrointestinal stromal tumors to neoadjuvant imatinib prior to successful surgical resection. Eur J Surg Oncol. 2014;40:420–8.
31. Eisenberg BL, Harris J, Blanke CD, Demetri GD, Heinrich MC, Watson JC, et al. Phase II trial of neoadjuvant/adjuvant imatinib mesylate (IM) for advanced primary and metastatic/recurrent operable gastrointestinal stromal tumor (GIST): early results of RTOG 0132/ACRIN 6665. J Surg Oncol. 2009;99:42–7.

32. Van den Abbeele AD, Gatsonis C, de Vries DJ, Melenevsky Y, Szot-Barnes A, Yap JT, et al. ACRIN 6665/RTOG 0132 phase II trial of neoadjuvant imatinib mesylate for operable malignant gastrointestinal stromal tumor: monitoring with 18F-FDG PET and correlation with genotype and GLUT4 expression. J Nucl Med. 2012;53:567–74.
33. Wang D, Zhang Q, Blanke CD, Demetri GD, Heinrich MC, Watson JC, et al. Phase II trial of neoadjuvant/adjuvant imatinib mesylate for advanced primary and metastatic/recurrent operable gastrointestinal stromal tumors: long-term follow-up results of Radiation Therapy Oncology Group 0132. Ann Surg Oncol. 2012;19:1074–80.
34. Kurokawa Y, Yang HK, Cho H, Ryu MH, Masuzawa T, Park SR, et al. Phase II study of neoadjuvant imatinib in large gastrointestinal stromal tumours of the stomach. Br J Cancer. 2017;117:25–32.
35. Demetri GD, Wang Y, Wehrle E, Racine A, Nikolova Z, Blanke CD, et al. Imatinib plasma levels are correlated with clinical benefit in patients with unresectable/metastatic gastrointestinal stromal tumors. J Clin Oncol. 2009;27:3141–7.
36. Maier J, Lange T, Kerle I, Specht K, Bruegel M, Wickenhauser C, et al. Detection of mutant free circulating tumor DNA in the plasma of patients with gastrointestinal stromal tumor harboring activating mutations of CKIT or PDGFRA. Clin Cancer Res. 2013;19:4854–67.
37. Yoo C, Ryu MH, Kang BW, Yoon SK, Ryoo BY, Chang HM, et al. Cross-sectional study of imatinib plasma trough levels in patients with advanced gastrointestinal stromal tumors: impact of gastrointestinal resection on exposure to imatinib. J Clin Oncol. 2010;28:1554–9.

New Agents for Gastrointestinal Stromal Tumors

11

Yoichi Naito and Toshihiko Doi

Abstract

Gastrointestinal stromal tumors (GISTs) are rare soft tissue sarcomas arising from gastrointestinal tract. Standard of care for metastatic GIST is molecular targeted therapy (imatinib, sunitinib, and regorafenib). Developmental therapeutics for GIST is focused on primary or acquired resistance to these agents. In this section, we discuss new agents for the treatment of GIST.

Keywords

Developmental therapeutics · Gastrointestinal stromal tumor · Imatinib resistance

Gastrointestinal stromal tumors (GISTs) are soft tissue sarcomas arising mainly from the gastrointestinal tract. In most cases, *KIT* or *PDGFRa* mutations are crucial for the development of the disease; thus, such genomic alterations could be the targets for treatment. GIST without *KIT*/*PDGFRa* mutations are called "wild-type GIST" and are usually resistant to the standard treatment for GIST with these mutations. Imatinib, sunitinib, and regorafenib are receptor tyrosine kinase inhibitors of KIT that have been approved for use worldwide. The efficacy and safety of these agents will be discussed elsewhere. Developmental therapeutics for GIST is focused on two domains: (1) overcoming resistance to imatinib and (2) novel agents for wild-type GIST. In this section, we discuss new agents for the treatment of GIST. Key phase II and III studies are listed in Table 11.1.

Y. Naito (✉) · T. Doi
Department of Experimental Therapeutics, National Cancer Center Hospital East, Kashiwa, Chiba, Japan
e-mail: ynaito@east.ncc.go.jp

Y. Kurokawa, Y. Komatsu (eds.), *Gastrointestinal Stromal Tumor*,
https://doi.org/10.1007/978-981-13-3206-7_11

Table 11.1 Key phase II and III studies for advanced GISTs (https://clinicaltrials.gov/, https://www.cancer.gov/publications/dictionaries/ accessed on June 20, 2018)

(a) Phase III studies

Drug	Explanation (NCI drug dictionary)	Registration	Trial
Avapritinib (BLU-285)	An orally bioavailable inhibitor of specific mutated forms of platelet-derived growth factor receptor alpha (PDGFR alpha; PDGFRa) and mast/stem cell factor receptor c-Kit (SCFR), with potential antineoplastic activity. Upon oral administration, BLU-285 specifically binds to and inhibits specific mutant forms of PDGFRa and c-Kit, including the PDGFRa D842V mutant and various *KIT* exon 17 mutants	NCT03465722	(VOYAGER) study of avapritinib vs regorafenib in patients with locally advanced unresectable or metastatic GIST
Crenolanib	An orally bioavailable benzimidazole targeting the platelet-derived growth factor receptor (PDGFR) subtypes alpha and beta and FMS-related tyrosine kinase 3 (Flt3), with potential antineoplastic activity	NCT02847429	Randomized trial of crenolanib in subjects with *D842V* mutated GIST
Retaspimycin (IPI-504)	The hydrochloride salt of a small-molecule inhibitor of heat shock protein 90 (HSP90) with antiproliferative and antineoplastic activities	NCT00688766	Study evaluating IPI-504 in patients with gastrointestinal stromal tumors (GIST) following failure of at least imatinib and sunitinib
Masitinib	Masitinib selectively binds to and inhibits both the wild-type and mutated forms of the stem cell factor receptor (c-Kit; *SCFR*); platelet-derived growth factor receptor (*PDGFR*); fibroblast growth factor receptor 3 (*FGFR3*); and, to a lesser extent, focal adhesion kinase (*FAK*)	NCT02009423	Masitinib vs. placebo—phase III study to compare the efficacy and safety of masitinib to placebo in patients with localized, primary GIST after complete surgery and with high risk of recurrence
		NCT01694277	A phase 3 study to evaluate efficacy and safety of masitinib in comparison to sunitinib in patients with gastrointestinal stromal tumor after progression with imatinib
		NCT00812240	A phase 3 study to evaluate efficacy and safety of masitinib in comparison to imatinib in patients with gastro-intestinal stromal tumor in first-line medical treatment

Table 11.1 (continued)

(a) Phase III studies			
Drug	Explanation (NCI drug dictionary)	Registration	Trial
L-carnitine	A dietary supplement containing the levo-enantiomers of carnitine and tartrate with potential chemoprotective and antioxidant activities	NCT03426722	L-carnitine vs. placebo for the treatment of muscle cramps after imatinib in gastrointestinal stromal tumors
DCC-2618	An orally bioavailable switch pocket control inhibitor of wild-type and mutated forms of the tumor-associated antigens (*TAA*) mast/stem cell factor receptor (*SCFR*) *KIT* and platelet-derived growth factor receptor alpha (PDGFR-alpha; *PDGFRa*), with potential antineoplastic activity. DCC-2618 also inhibits several other kinases, including vascular endothelial growth factor receptor type 2 (VEGFR2; KDR), angiopoietin-1 receptor (TIE2; TEK), PDGFR-beta, and macrophage colony-stimulating factor 1 receptor (FMS; CSF1R)	NCT03353753	Phase 3 study of DCC-2618 vs placebo in advanced GIST patients who have been treated with prior anticancer therapies
Bevacizumab	A recombinant humanized monoclonal antibody directed against the vascular endothelial growth factor (VEGF)	NCT00324987	Imatinib mesylate with or without bevacizumab in treating patients with metastatic or unresectable gastrointestinal stromal tumor
(b) Phase II studies			
Drug	*Explanation (NCI)*	*Registration*	*Trial*
Epacadostat, pembrolizumab	An orally available hydroxyamidine and inhibitor of indoleamine 2,3-dioxygenase (IDO1), with potential immunomodulating and antineoplastic activities	NCT03291054	Epacadostat and pembrolizumab in patients with GIST
Olaratumab	A fully human IgG1 monoclonal antibody directed against platelet-derived growth factor receptor alpha (PDGFR alpha) with potential antineoplastic activity	NCT01316263	A study of olaratumab (IMC-3G3) in previously treated participants with unresectable and/or metastatic gastrointestinal stromal tumors
Perifosine	An orally active alkyl-phosphocholine compound with potential antineoplastic activity It acts as an Akt and PI3K inhibitor	NCT00455559	Phase II study of perifosine plus Gleevec for patients with GIST

(continued)

Table 11.1 (continued)

(a) Phase III studies

Drug	Explanation (NCI drug dictionary)	Registration	Trial
Famitinib	Famitinib binds to and inhibits several RTKs dysregulated in a variety of tumors, including stem cell factor receptor (c-Kit; SCFR), vascular endothelial growth factor receptor (VEGFR) 2 and 3, platelet-derived growth factor receptor (PDGFR), and FMS-like tyrosine kinases Flt1 and Flt3	NCT02336724	A study of famitinib in patients with gastrointestinal stromal tumor
Temozolomide	A triazene analog of dacarbazine with antineoplastic activity. As a cytotoxic alkylating agent, temozolomide is converted at physiologic pH to the short-lived active compound, monomethyl triazeno imidazole carboxamide (MTIC)	NCT00005597	S9926 temozolomide in patients with unresectable/metastatic gastrointestinal stromal tumors
Motesanib	The orally bioavailable diphosphate salt of a multiple-receptor tyrosine kinase inhibitor with potential antineoplastic activity. Motesanib selectively targets and inhibits vascular endothelial growth factor (VEGFR), platelet-derived growth factor (PDGFR), kit, and ret receptors, thereby inhibiting angiogenesis and cellular proliferation	NCT00254267	Evaluate the efficacy of AMG 706 to treat advanced gastrointestinal stromal tumors
		NCT00089960	Study of AMG 706 in subjects with advanced gastrointestinal stromal tumors (GISTs)
Nivolumab, Ipilimumab	A fully human immunoglobulin (Ig) G4 monoclonal antibody directed against the negative immunoregulatory human cell surface receptor programmed death-1 (PD-1, PCD-1,) with immune checkpoint inhibitory and antineoplastic activities	NCT02880020	Nivolumab with or without ipilimumab in treating patients with gastrointestinal stromal tumor that is metastatic or cannot be removed by surgery
Masitinib	Masitinib selectively binds to and inhibits both the wild-type and mutated forms of the stem cell factor receptor (c-Kit; SCFR); platelet-derived growth factor receptor (PDGFR); fibroblast growth factor receptor 3 (FGFR3); and, to a lesser extent, focal adhesion kinase (FAK)	NCT01506336	A phase 2 study to evaluate efficacy and safety of masitinib in comparison to sunitinib in patients with gastro-intestinal stromal tumor resistant to imatinib

Table 11.1 (continued)

(a) Phase III studies

Drug	Explanation (NCI drug dictionary)	Registration	Trial
Luminespib (AUY922)	A derivative of 4,5-diarylisoxazole and a third-generation heat shock protein 90 (Hsp90) inhibitor with potential antineoplastic activity	NCT01404650	Study of Hsp90 inhibitor AUY922 for the treatment of patients with refractory gastrointestinal stromal tumor
BBI503	An orally available cancer cell stemness kinase inhibitor with potential antineoplastic activity. Although the exact target has not been fully elucidated, BBI503 targets and inhibits one or more pathways involved in cancer stem cell survival	NCT02232620	A study of BBI503 in adult patients with advanced gastrointestinal stromal tumors
Palbociclib	An orally available cyclin-dependent kinase (CDK) inhibitor with potential antineoplastic activity. Palbociclib selectively inhibits cyclin-dependent kinase 4 (CDK4) and 6 (CDK6), thereby inhibiting retinoblastoma (Rb) protein phosphorylation early in the G1 phase, leading to cell cycle arrest	NCT01907607	Efficacy and safety of PD-0332991 in patients with advanced gastrointestinal stromal tumors refractory to imatinib and sunitinib
XL820	XL820 binds to and inhibits the receptor tyrosine kinases for vascular endothelial growth factor (VEGF), c-kit, and platelet-derived growth factor (PDGF)	NCT00570635	A phase 2 study of XL820 in adults with advanced GIST resistant to imatinib and/or sunitinib
Cediranib	Competing with adenosine triphosphate, cediranib binds to and inhibits all three vascular endothelial growth factor receptor (VEGFR-1, -2, -3) tyrosine kinases, thereby blocking VEGF-signaling, angiogenesis, and tumor cell growth	NCT00385203	The biological activity of cediranib (AZD2171) in gastro-intestinal stromal tumors (GISTs)
Oblimersen	Oblimersen inhibits Bcl-2 mRNA translation, which may result in decreased expression of the Bcl-2 protein and tumor cell apoptosis. This agent may enhance the efficacy of standard cytotoxic chemotherapy	NCT00091078	Oblimersen and imatinib mesylate in treating patients with advanced gastrointestinal stromal tumors that cannot be removed by surgery

(continued)

Table 11.1 (continued)

(a) Phase III studies			
Drug	Explanation (NCI drug dictionary)	Registration	Trial
Paclitaxel	Paclitaxel binds to tubulin and inhibits the disassembly of microtubules, thereby resulting in the inhibition of cell division	NCT02607332	A trial of paclitaxel in patients with metastatic or advanced gastrointestinal stromal tumors (GIST) after failure to imatinib and sunitinib
Guadecitabine	A dinucleotide antimetabolite of a decitabine linked via a phosphodiester bond to a guanosine, with potential antineoplastic activity. Following metabolic activation by phosphorylation and incorporation into DNA, guadecitabine inhibits DNA methyltransferase, thereby causing genome-wide and non-specific hypomethylation and inducing S-phase cell cycle arrest	NCT03165721	A phase II trial of the DNA methyl transferase inhibitor, guadecitabine (SGI-110), in children and adults with wild-type GIST, pheochromocytoma and paraganglioma associated with succinate dehydrogenase deficiency and HLRCC-associated kidney cancer
Vatalanib	An orally bioavailable anilinophthalazine with potential antineoplastic activity. Vatalanib binds to and inhibits the protein kinase domain of vascular endothelial growth factor receptors 1 and 2; both receptor tyrosine kinases are involved in angiogenesis. This agent also binds to and inhibits related receptor tyrosine kinases, including platelet-derived growth factor (PDGF) receptor, c-kit, and c-Fms	NCT00117299	PTK787/ZK222584 in the treatment of metastatic gastrointestinal stromal tumors resistant to imatinib
Linsitinib	An orally bioavailable small molecule inhibitor of the insulin-like growth factor 1 receptor (IGF-1R) with potential antineoplastic activity. Linsitinib selectively inhibits IGF-1R, which may result in the inhibition of tumor cell proliferation and the induction of tumor cell apoptosis	NCT01560260	Linsitinib in treating patients with gastrointestinal stromal tumors

Table 11.1 (continued)

(a) Phase III studies			
Drug	Explanation (NCI drug dictionary)	Registration	Trial
Selumetinib	Selumetinib is an ATP-independent inhibitor of mitogen-activated protein kinase kinase (MEK or MAPK/ERK kinase) 1 and 2	NCT03109301	Mitogen activated protein kinase kinase (MEK1/2) inhibitor selumetinib (AZD6244 hydrogen Sulfate) in people with neurofibromatosis type 1 (NF1) mutated gastrointestinal stromal tumors (GIST)
Temsirolimus	An ester analog of rapamycin. Temsirolimus binds to and inhibits the mammalian target of rapamycin (mTOR), resulting in decreased expression of mRNAs necessary for cell cycle progression and arresting cells in the G1 phase of the cell cycle	NCT00087074	CCI-779 in treating patients with soft tissue sarcoma or gastrointestinal stromal tumor

11.1 Resistance to Imatinib

Approximately 70% of imatinib-resistant GISTs harbor acquired mutations in *KIT*. Data suggest that secondary mutations occur mainly in exon 13, 14 (ATP-binding pocket), or 17 (activation loop) of *KIT* (Fig. 11.1) [1]. Novel KIT inhibitors are currently under investigation.

11.2 Avapritinib (BLU-285)

Avapritinib (Blueprint Medicines, Cambridge, Massachusetts) is an oral investigational drug that is potent and is a selective, small-molecule inhibitor of KIT (Table 11.2) [1]. The phase I "NAVIGATOR" study has been completed for patients with *PDGFR D842V*-mutated GIST, but it is ongoing for patients with *KIT*- or *PDGFRa*-mutated GIST after receiving imatinib [2]. At the 2017 Congress of American Society of Clinical Oncology, preliminary results of 40 patients with GIST (21 *PDGFRa* mutant/19 *KIT* mutant) treated with BLU-285 at doses ranging from 30 to 600 mg were reported. Of 17 patients with *PDGFRα D842V*, 7 had a confirmed partial response (PR) (overall response rate [ORR], 41%) and 10 had

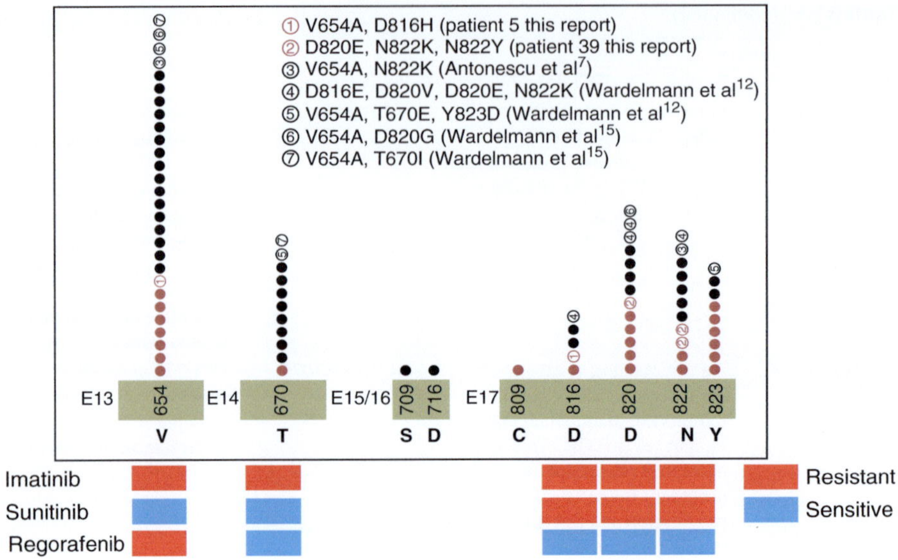

Fig. 11.1 Secondary *KIT* mutations

Table 11.2 Potential activities of KIT inhibitors

Compound	Inhibitor type	KIT WT IC50 N (nM)	KIT del557–558 exon 11 IC50 (nM)	KIT D816V exon 17 IC50 (nM)	PDGFRA D842V exon 18 IC50 (nM)
BLU-285	Type I	73	0.6	0.27	0.24
Imatinib	Type II	261	12	8150	759
Sunitinib	Type II	37	7	207	120
Regorafenib	Type II	204	17	3640	810
Crenolanib	Type I	36	2.1	1.5	0.2
Midostaurin	Type I	26	2.2	2.9	4.9

stable disease (SD). Of 11 patients with *KIT* mutations, 2 had a PR (ORR, 18%) and 5 had SD. Adverse events of avapritinib are mainly gastrointestinal disorders and periorbital edema. Hand–foot syndrome was not reported in this study. Up to 30% of patients experienced dose-dependent cognitive symptoms, mostly grade 1 or 2. A randomized phase III "VOYAGER" trial designed to explore the safety and efficacy of avapritinib compared to those of regorafenib in patients with advanced GIST who have progressed to receive imatinib is currently underway [3].

11.3 DCC-2618

DCC-2618 (Deciphera) is a pan-KIT and PDGFRa kinase switch control inhibitor resilient to de-novo and drug resistance mutations and with a potency independent of ATP concentration. Janku and colleagues reported a phase I dose-escalation study of oral DCC-2618 at doses ranging from 40 mg up to 400 mg [4]. Of the 37 evaluable patients, 5 achieved a PR (14%). Fourteen (58%) of the 24 evaluable patients receiving DCC-2618 at doses of 100 mg/day showed progression-free survival (PFS) lasting more than 6 months. Toxicities of grade 3 or higher in the study ($n = 70$) included anemia in 19 patients, asymptomatic lipase increase in 13, hypertension in 6, elevated creatinine phosphokinase in 2, and increased unconjugated bilirubin in 2 patients. Currently, a phase III study is underway to compare the efficacy of DCC-2618 with that of placebo in patients who have received prior imatinib, sunitinib, and regorafenib treatment [5]. Moreover, a phase III study for the second-line treatment of GIST is planned (https://www.deciphera.com/pipeline/dcc-2618/. Accessed 20 June 2018).

11.4 Masitinib

Masitinib (AB Science) is a novel oral inhibitor of both KIT and PDGFRA receptors. In a phase II study evaluating masitinib as the first-line treatment for advanced GIST, the ORR was 53.3% and the estimated median PFS was 41.3 months [6]. Another randomized phase II study evaluating masitinib after failure of imatinib showed a median PFS of 3.71 months and a significantly lower occurrence of severe adverse events than with sunitinib use [7]. Nausea/vomiting was the only toxicity more frequently observed in the masitinib arm than in the sunitinib arm. Three phase III trials are currently ongoing, the first comparing masitinib with sunitinib in patients with advanced/recurrent imatinib-resistant GIST [8], the second comparing masitinib with imatinib as the first-line therapy for patients with advanced GIST [9], and the third comparing masitinib with a placebo in the adjuvant setting for high-risk patients with resected GIST [10].

11.5 Heat Shock Protein (HSP)90 Inhibitors

HSP90 is a protein chaperone that maintains proper folding, function, and stability of key oncoproteins including KIT. The use of first-generation HSP90 inhibitors in patients with advanced tumors is limited because of hepatotoxicity. Retaspimycin (or IPI-504; Infinity Pharmaceuticals) is a novel HSP90 inhibitor that is highly water soluble. In a phase I study, retaspimycin showed promising activity, with a disease control rate (DCR) of 73% and acceptable toxicity [11]. However, the confirmatory phase III "RING" trial was terminated early because of the high occurrence of hepatotoxicity and treatment-related death [12]. Luminespib (or AUY922; Vernalis) is another HSP90 inhibitor. A phase II study of luminespib was reported; however, the study was stopped early because of slow accrual [13]. The median PFS was 3.9 months and the clinical benefit rate was 64%. TAS-116 is an oral non-ansamycin, non-purine, non-resorcinol, highly selective inhibitor of HSP90. Recently the results of a phase II study were reported [14]. The DCR was 85.0% ($n = 40$) and the median PFS was 4.4 months. A confirmatory phase III study is planned.

11.6 Targeting PDGFRA D842V

11.6.1 Crenolanib

Crenolanib (ARO-002 or CP-868,596; AROG Pharmaceuticals LLC) is a potent and selective inhibitor of t FLT3, PDGFRα, and PDGFRβ; however, crenolanib is relatively insensitive towards wild-type KIT. Nevertheless, homology considerations suggest that crenolanib could display clinically meaningful sensitivity against mutant-KIT isoforms [15]. A phase I/II study evaluated crenolanib in patients with PDGFRA D842V mutant GIST and reported a clinical benefit rate of 31% (5/16 patients) [16]. A phase III study (CRENOGIST) comparing crenolanib with placebo in patients with advanced or metastatic GIST with a D842V mutation in *PDGFRA* is currently underway [17].

11.7 Wild-Type GIST and Miscellaneous

Approximately 10% of GISTs lack *KIT* or *PDGFRA* mutations; such tumors are called "wild-type GIST." Among them, the *RAF-RAS-MAPK* pathway abnormalities such as *BRAF* V600E, *HRAS*, *NRAS*, or *NF-1* mutations, and succinate dehydrogenase (*SDH*) deficiency have been detected [18]. Gene fusions involving *FGFR* and *NTRK* are rarely detected [19]. Imatinib is not active against *SDH*-mutant GIST because of the lack of an active *KIT* mutation [20]. The glutaminase inhibitor CB-8 [21] and the DNA methyltransferase inhibitor guadecitabine (SGI-110) have been investigated and the results of these investigations are awaited [22]. For patients with GIST and an *NF-1* mutation, the MEK inhibitor selumetinib has been investigated [23]. The BRAF inhibitor dabrafenib showed prolonged antitumor activity in patients with *BRAF* V600E-mutated GIST [24]. NTRK fusions are rare; however, initial success with TRK inhibitors has been reported. TRK inhibitors larotrectinib (LOXO-101) [25] and entrectinib (RXDX-101) [26] have been suggested for patients with GIST and NTRK fusions.

Immune checkpoint inhibitors have been approved worldwide for the treatment of a variety of solid tumors such as malignant melanoma, non-small cell lung cancer, and renal cell carcinoma [27]. Unfortunately, the efficacy of these inhibitors for GIST is limited. A randomized phase II study of nivolumab alone and in combination with ipilimumab was reported [28]. In the nivolumab-only arm, 3/7 patients had SD, with a CBR of 42.8%. The median PFS was 8 weeks. In the nivolumab plus ipilimumab arm, 1/5 (20%) patients had a PR and 1/5 had SD for a CBR of 40%. The median PFS of the combination arm was 8.43 weeks.

11.8 Conclusion

Imatinib, sunitinib, and regorafenib are active against GISTs; however, the prognosis of advanced GIST is not satisfactory. Novel KIT inhibitors such as avapritinib, DCC-2618, and masitinib are currently under investigation. GISTs without *KIT* and

PDGFRA mutations might harbor RAS-RAF-MAPK pathway alterations, SDH deficiency, FGFR fusions, or NTRK fusions. Targeting of these abnormalities is currently underway.

References

1. Evans EK, Gardino AK, Kim JL, Hodous BL, Shutes A, Davis A, Zhu XJ, Schmidt-Kittler O, Wilson D, Wilson K, DiPietro L, Zhang Y, Brooijmans N, LaBranche TP, Wozniak A, Gebreyohannes YK, Schöffski P, Heinrich MC, DeAngelo DJ, Miller S, Wolf B, Kohl N, Guzi T, Lydon N, Boral A, Lengauer C. A precision therapy against cancers driven by KIT/PDGFRA mutations. Sci Transl Med. 2017;9(414):eaao1690.
2. Heinrich MC, Jones RL, von Mehren M, Schoffski P, Bauer S, Mir O, Cassier PA, Eskens F, Shi H, Alvarez-Diez T, Schmidt-Kittler O, Healy ME, Wolf BB, George S. Clinical activity of BLU-285 in advanced gastrointestinal stromal tumor (GIST). J Clin Oncol. 2017;35(15_suppl):11011.
3. (VOYAGER) Study of avapritinib vs regorafenib in patients with locally advanced unresectable or metastatic GIST. Available from https://clinicaltrials.gov/ct2/show/NCT03465722.
4. Janku F, et al. Encouraging activity of novel pan-KIT and PDGFRα inhibitor DCC-2618 in patients (pts) with gastrointestinal stromal tumor (GIST). Ann Oncol. 2017;28(5):v521–38.
5. Phase 3 study of DCC-2618 vs placebo in advanced GIST patients who have been treated with prior anticancer therapies (invictus). Available from https://clinicaltrials.gov/ct2/show/NCT03353753.
6. Le Cesne A, Blay JY, Bui BN, Bouché O, Adenis A, Domont J, Cioffi A, Ray-Coquard I, Lassau N, Bonvalot S, Moussy A, Kinet JP, Hermine O. Phase II study of oral masitinib mesylate in imatinib-naïve patients with locally advanced or metastatic gastro-intestinal stromal tumour (GIST). Eur J Cancer. 2010;46(8):1344–51.
7. Adenis A, Blay JY, Bui-Nguyen B, Bouché O, Bertucci F, Isambert N, Bompas E, Chaigneau L, Domont J, Ray-Coquard I, Blésius A, Van Tine BA, Bulusu VR, Dubreuil P, Mansfield CD, Acin Y, Moussy A, Hermine O, Le Cesne A. Masitinib in advanced gastrointestinal stromal tumor (GIST) after failure of imatinib: a randomized controlled open-label trial. Ann Oncol. 2014;25(9):1762–9.
8. A phase 3 study to evaluate efficacy and safety of masitinib in comparison to sunitinib in patients with gastrointestinal stromal tumour after progression with imatinib. Available from https://clinicaltrials.gov/ct2/show/NCT01694277.
9. A phase 3 study to evaluate efficacy and safety of masitinib in comparison to imatinib in patients with gastro-intestinal stromal tumour in first line medical treatment. Available from https://clinicaltrials.gov/ct2/show/NCT00812240.
10. Masitinib vs placebo - phase iii study to compare the efficacy and safety of masitinib to placebo in patients with localized, primary gist after complete surgery and with high risk of recurrence. Available from https://clinicaltrials.gov/ct2/show/NCT02009423.
11. Wagner AJ, Chugh R, Rosen LS, Morgan JA, George S, Gordon M, Dunbar J, Normant E, Grayzel D, Demetri GD. A phase I study of the HSP90 inhibitor retaspimycin hydrochloride (IPI-504) in patients with gastrointestinal stromal tumors or soft-tissue sarcomas. Clin Cancer Res. 2013;19(21):6020–9.
12. Demetri G, Le Cesne A, Von Mehren M, Chmielowski B, Bauer S, Chow W, et al. Final results from a phase III study of IPI-504 (retaspimycin hydrochloride) versus placebo in patients (pts) with gastrointestinal stromal tumors (GIST) following failure of kinase inhibitor therapies. 2010 ASCO Gastrointestinal Cancers Symposium. Abstract No. 64.
13. Bendell JC, Bauer TM, Lamar R, Joseph M, Penley W, Thompson DS, Spigel DR, Owera R, Lane CM, Earwood C, Burris HA 3rd. A phase 2 study of the Hsp90 inhibitor AUY922 as treatment for patients with refractory gastrointestinal stromal tumors. Cancer Investig. 2016;34(6):265–70.

14. Kurokawa Y, Doi T, Sawaki A, Komatsu Y, Ozaka M, Takahashi T, Naito Y, Okubo S, Nishida T. Phase II study of TAS-116, an oral inhibitor of heat shock protein 90 (HSP90) in metastatic or unresectable gastrointestinal stromal tumor refractory to imatinib, sunitinib and regorafenib. Ann Oncol. 2017;28(Suppl 5):Abstr 1479PD.
15. Kampa-Schittenhelm KM, Frey J, Haeusser LA, Illing B, Pavlovsky AA, Blumenstock G, Schittenhelm MM. Crenolanib is a type I tyrosine kinase inhibitor that inhibits mutant KIT D816 isoforms prevalent in systemic mastocytosis and core binding factor leukemia. Oncotarget. 2017;8(47):82897–909.
16. von Mehren M, Tetzlaff ED, Macaraeg M, Davis J, Agarwal V, Ramachandran A, et al. Dose escalating study of crenolanib besylate in advanced GIST patients with PDGFRA D842V activating mutations. J Clin Oncol. 2016;34(suppl 5):11010.
17. Randomized trial of crenolanib in subjects with D842V mutated GIST. Available from https://clinicaltrials.gov/ct2/show/NCT02847429.
18. Corless CL, Barnett CM, Heinrich MC. Gastrointestinal stromal tumours: origin and molecular oncology. Nat Rev Cancer. 2011;11(12):865–78.
19. Shi E, Chmielecki J, Tang CM, Wang K, Heinrich MC, Kang G, Corless CL, Hong D, Fero KE, Murphy JD, Fanta PT, Ali SM, De Siena M, Burgoyne AM, Movva S, Madlensky L, Heestand GM, Trent JC, Kurzrock R, Morosini D, Ross JS, Harismendy O, Sicklick JK. FGFR1 and NTRK3 actionable alterations in "Wild-Type" gastrointestinal stromal tumors. J Transl Med. 2016;14(1):339.
20. Miettinen M, Wang ZF, Sarlomo-Rikala M, Osuch C, Rutkowski P, Lasota J. Succinate dehydrogenase-deficient GISTs: a clinicopathologic, immunohistochemical, and molecular genetic study of 66 gastric GISTs with predilection to young age. Am J Surg Pathol. 2011;35(11):1712–21.
21. Study of the glutaminase inhibitor CB-839 in solid tumors. Available from https://clinicaltrials.gov/ct2/show/NCT02071862.
22. A phase II trial of the DNA methyl transferase inhibitor, guadecitabine (SGI-110), in children and adults with wild type GIST, pheochromocytoma and paraganglioma associated with succinate dehydrogenase deficiency and HLRCC-associated kidney cancer. Available from https://clinicaltrials.gov/ct2/show/NCT03165721.
23. Mitogen activated protein kinase kinase (MEK1/2) inhibitor selumetinib (AZD6244 Hydrogen Sulfate) in people with neurofibromatosis type 1 (NF1) mutated gastrointestinal stromal tumors (GIST). Available from https://clinicaltrials.gov/ct2/show/NCT03109301.
24. Falchook GS, Trent JC, Heinrich MC, Beadling C, Patterson J, Bastida CC, et al. BRAF mutant gastrointestinal stromal tumor: first report of regression with BRAF inhibitor dabrafenib (GSK2118436) and whole exomic sequencing for analysis of acquired resistance. Oncotarget. 2013;4(2):310–5.
25. Drilon A, Laetsch TW, Kummar S, DuBois SG, Lassen UN, Demetri GD, Nathenson M, Doebele RC, Farago AF, Pappo AS, Turpin B, Dowlati A, Brose MS, Mascarenhas L, Federman N, Berlin J, El-Deiry WS, Baik C, Deeken J, Boni V, Nagasubramanian R, Taylor M, Rudzinski ER, Meric-Bernstam F, Sohal DPS, Ma PC, Raez LE, Hechtman JF, Benayed R, Ladanyi M, Tuch BB, Ebata K, Cruickshank S, Ku NC, Cox MC, Hawkins DS, Hong DS, Hyman DM. Efficacy of larotrectinib in TRK fusion-positive cancers in adults and children. N Engl J Med. 2018;378(8):731–9.
26. Liu D, Offin M, Harnicar S, Li BT, Drilon A. Entrectinib: an orally available, selective tyrosine kinase inhibitor for the treatment of NTRK, ROS1, and ALK fusion-positive solid tumors. Ther Clin Risk Manag. 2018;14:1247–52.
27. Hargadon KM, Johnson CE, Williams CJ. Immune checkpoint blockade therapy for cancer: an overview of FDA-approved immune checkpoint inhibitors. Int Immunopharmacol. 2018;62:29–39.
28. Singh AS, Chmielowski B, Randolph Hecht J, Rosen LS, Wang X, Brackert S, Adame CR, Linares PJ, Schink E, Marubio LM, Eilber FC. A randomized phase 2 study of nivolumab monotherapy versus nivolumab combined with ipilimumab in patients with metastatic or unresectable gastrointestinal stromal tumor (GIST). J Clin Oncol. 2018;36(suppl 4S):abstr 55.

MIX
Papier aus verantwortungsvollen Quellen
Paper from responsible sources
FSC® C105338
FSC
www.fsc.org

If you have any concerns about our products,
you can contact us on
ProductSafety@springernature.com

In case Publisher is established outside the EU,
the EU authorized representative is:
Springer Nature Customer Service Center GmbH
Europaplatz 3, 69115 Heidelberg, Germany

Printed by Libri Plureos GmbH
in Hamburg, Germany